SIMPLY PAINTING

WATERCOLOURS BOOK 2

PICTURES ANYONE CAN PAINT WITH WATERCOLOURS

Frank Clarke

Published by

 ART GALLERY

Dedication

This book is dedicated to Having Some More Fun with a paint brush.

Appreciation

My thanks goes to all the people who have written to me with such kind words, but for them this book would never have been possible. Thank you for helping me to fulfil a dream - to tell the world about the wonderful hobby of painting.

I must not forget Terri who amazed me by being able to unscramble my handwriting.

Contents

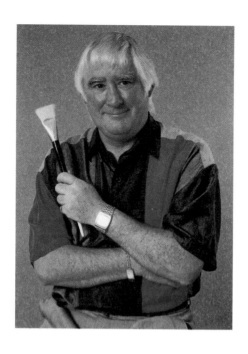

Frank Clarke

Born in Dublin, Ireland, Frank Clarke began painting just 15 years ago and has since become one of Ireland's most well known and sought after artists.

During this time, Frank developed his artistic talents and a unique approach to painting which he calls **Have Some More Fun**. A natural teacher, Frank is convinced that **anyone can paint** and has travelled the world sharing his **Simply Painting** technique with a wide audience of young and old alike.

Using this method Frank has introduced thousands of people to the basics of watercolours and acrylics, the fun of painting, and the realisation that 'anyone who can draw the letter M can paint'.

While painting now plays an important role in his life and has grown to include books, videos, television series and painting kits, he enjoys it so much that he still regards it as his, 'hobby gone mad'.

With several successful television series screening on stations in the United States, United Kingdom and his native Ireland, Frank brings his skill, enthusiasm, and entertaining style to everyone, to encourage, inspire, and instruct them how to paint.

In this book, Frank is eager to share his hobby with you in his own relaxed and witty manner.

Introduction

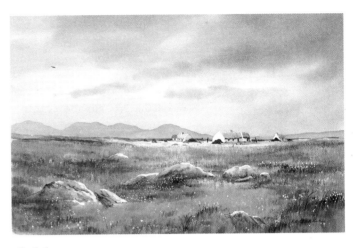

When my publishers asked me to write another watercolour book my first reaction was 'I can't', but the funny thing was, once I started my head flooded with ideas. I became so enthused that I stayed at my desk for hours making notes. The following pages are the fruits of those deliberations.

Firstly, most of the requests I receive are for more pictures to paint and how to paint them. With that in mind I have produced seven different subjects for you to paint. The lessons are in the same format as my first watercolour book *Simply Painting* **Watercolours** 'Teaches anyone to Paint' which I hope you have read.

Using my **Have Some More Fun** system I believe *anyone can paint*. I just ask that you read this book up to the first lesson before you start and you will soon realise I am correct in what I say. It won't take long and I promise it will be time well spent. It will explain the materials you require, how to use them and also, how my **Have Some More Fun** method works and believe me it works, I have never had a failure. So get yourself into a comfy corner and off you go.

Like any hobby someone has to show you how to start and that's where Mr. Brush and myself come in. Most art books start by assuming you have some prior knowledge of how to paint. This is because they are written for the leisure painter who can already paint, in the belief that the only people who buy art books are people who can already paint. This represents about 3% of the population. WHAT ABOUT THE OTHER 97%?

I want to show everyone how to start painting and to do that I believe one must feel, 'I can do that'. Indeed there are many leisure painters who are still not sure if they are on the right track. I know, I muddled around for quite some time myself when I first started to paint. In fact I have one of my first paintings framed and hanging in my studio. When I painted it I was pleased but my wife Peg said, 'It looks more like an elephant with its feet up in the air than a forest scene.' But then I did not have the benefit of anyone to show me how to START.

Let me tell you something about this wonderful hobby. You do not have to start off painting pictures like the Impressionists or Constable or Turner, you can start with simple pictures and it's up to you how far you want to advance. Every hour you spend enjoying your hobby will make you a better painter. By knowing how to start you will be able to enjoy your painting from the first picture.

I have received many thousands of letters and they all have one theme, 'You got me started and I love it'. These letters are from people of all ages, from 5 to 95 years. In fact, in one of my classes I had a lady beginner who was 95 years old and she was terrific, so you see age is no barrier.

There is another aspect to painting which will add to your enjoyment. You will begin to have an interest in how the great artists painted their masterpieces and will want to see their works. When you visit art galleries you will be able to see the methods used by these artists and understand them, because you will be doing the same.

What you are getting is a crash course in art appreciation and you know it's very difficult to appreciate something if you don't understand it. So before you start let me say, 'I will show you how to ride the bicycle, it's up to you what direction you take.' You may in time prefer to paint flowers, still life or figures, that's up to you.

So once again let me introduce you good friend Mr. Brush who will help guide you through this book.

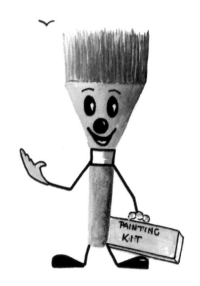

1: Materials

Paints

Watercolour paints come in two forms, tubes and pans. Tubes contain moist paint ready for use. Pans are blocks of paint which you soften with water first, just like the ones in a child's paint box.

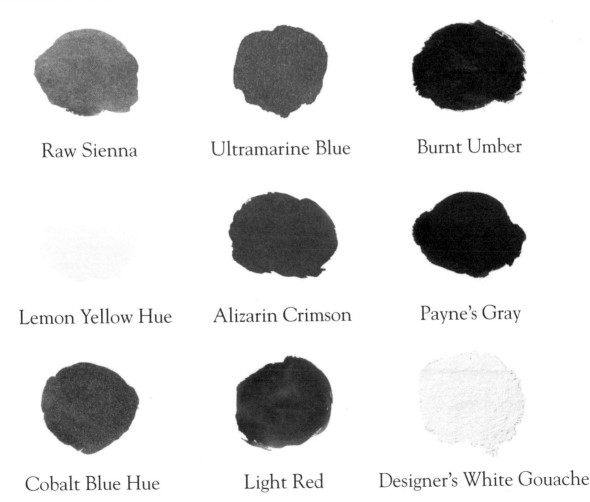

I recommend Winsor & Newton Cotman watercolours in tubes. They are student's quality and less expensive. I use them myself and I find them excellent. You will also need a tube of Winsor & Newton Designer's Permanent White Gouache or if you can't get White Gouache, a tube of Chinese White watercolour paint will do.

The colours we need are:

Raw Sienna   Ultramarine Blue   Burnt Umber

Lemon Yellow Hue   Alizarin Crimson   Payne's Gray

Cobalt Blue Hue   Light Red   Designer's White Gouache

For the lessons in this book we use only eight different tubes of paint because with this selection you will be able to mix all the colours you require.

You will notice there are two blues and no green. This is because we can make our own green using one of the blues and Lemon Yellow Hue. Ultramarine Blue is a darker blue and there is more red in it than Cobalt Blue Hue. So mixing Ultramarine Blue with Lemon Yellow Hue will make a green. If you want a different green just mix Cobalt Blue Hue with Lemon Yellow Hue.

I always put out the paints as I use them. I don't see any sense in laying out all the paints and filling the palette with paint I may not use. However it is a funny thing about artists, we are generous in many ways, but we can be very mean with paint. I've been to art classes where you'd ask another artist for some paint and you would think you were asking them for their house. Yet the very same people would wine and dine you, but don't ask them for a penny worth of paint. Don't be mean with the paint when you put it out.

Tip: When you put the paints on the palette, remember to put the tops back on the tubes.

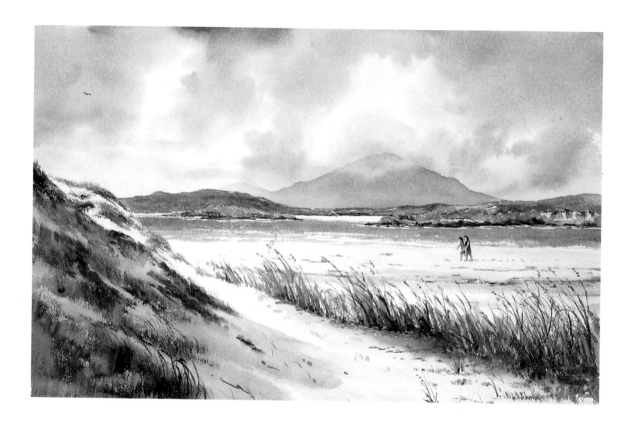

Brushes

To paint the pictures in this book you will only need two brushes, one large and one small.

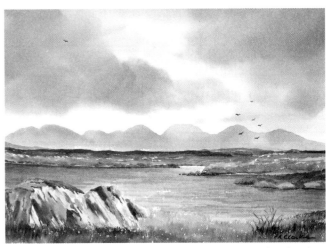

Let's start with the **Simply Painting** Large Brush which is a 1.5"(38mm) goat hair brush. It took me many months to devise this brush and get it to act as I wanted. In fact my studio was covered in goat hair and dissected brushes. However I feel the outcome was worth the effort.

The small brush I recommend is my **Simply Painting** No. 3 Rigger. Both brushes are manufactured by Winsor & Newton, as indeed is the **Simply Painting Watercolour** Painting Set.

As I have often said, if you don't have these brushes it does not preclude you from painting. You can use any large and small watercolour brush, although it does help to use the recommended brushes.

When buying brushes don't be afraid to ask for help in the store. You may find cheap imitation brushes but be careful they may turn out to be a waste of your good money. To give the best results the large brush should be made of goat hair.

When you first use new brushes it is not uncommon for some hairs to fall out. Don't worry just leave them there and you can blow them away when the picture dries. If you try to pick them off you may damage your watercolour paper.

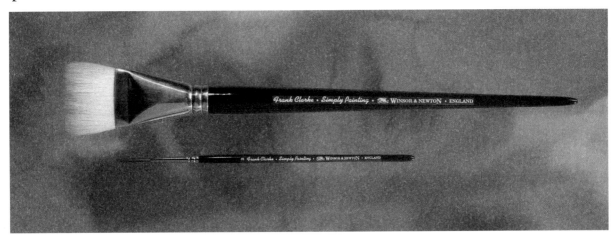

Paper

When painting with watercolours it is important to use <u>watercolour paper</u>. This is because it is specially made to absorb water and hold the pigment. It is available with several surfaces and comes in many weights or thicknesses. These weights range from 90 lbs (190gsm) to 400 lbs (900gsm) and the higher the weight the thicker the paper. There are three principal surfaces available, Hot Pressed which is smooth, Not or Cold Pressed which is semi-rough, and Rough. Watercolour paper is obtainable in large sheets or in pads which are cut to standard sizes.

The size of pictures we're going to paint is 14" x 10" (35cm x 25cm). I often use a sheet which is larger than this and rule out an area of 14" x 10" on it, then I can use the sides for doodling on. However, if you buy your pads exactly 14" x 10", you can use a spare sheet to test your paints on.

The paper I recommend for these lessons has a semi-rough or Not surface and is 140 lbs (300gsm) in weight or thickness. It is manufactured by Winsor & Newton and available from art stores.

Tip: If you are using a watercolour pad it is a good idea to tear the page from the pad and attach it to your board before you start to paint, otherwise some of the paint may spill over onto the next page and ruin it on you.

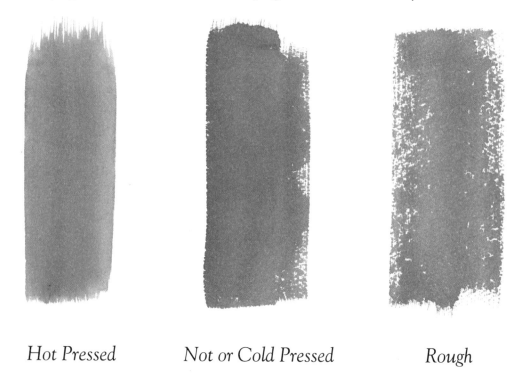

Hot Pressed   Not or Cold Pressed   Rough

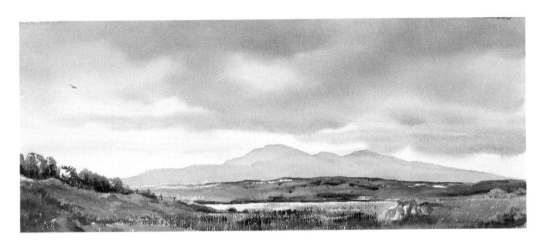

Palette

A palette is simply for holding and mixing paint and can be any large plate or tray provided it is white (it's easier to see the colours if it's white).

Just for your information you may read that an artist's palette is the colours he uses. Well this is also correct, a palette can be the colours an artist uses but when I refer to your palette I mean something to hold and mix your paint on.

Tip: Avoid using palettes which look like egg-trays.

Board

To paint watercolours it is necessary to place the paper on a firm surface, so you will need a board. A piece of hardboard or plywood will do fine as long as it's large enough. It needs to measure approximately 20" x 16" (50 x 40cm). If you can't find a piece around the house your local hardware store can provide you with something suitable.

You can become very attached to this piece of equipment. My board, which is just a piece hardboard, is about ten years old and on one occasion I drove forty miles back to a hotel to retrieve my beloved board which had only cost me pennies.

To use the board to best effect, raise the back of the board about 2" off the table by putting something under it.

If you happen to have an easel you can use it to support your board. I could ramble on about easels but I think it is suffice to say if you have one by all means use it. However it's not an essential part of watercolour equipment. If you do feel you require an easel make sure you obtain a watercolour easel.

Masking Fluid

Masking fluid is a latex rubber. It is available in bottles and can be obtained in most good art stores. It is manufactured in two formats, coloured and colourless.

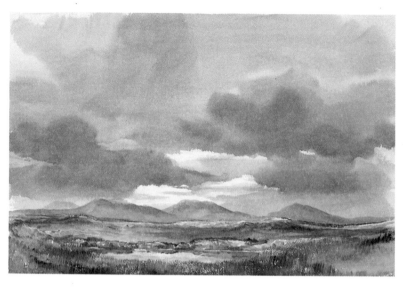

Both work well, however the coloured masking fluid (it's yellow) allows you to see more easily where it has been applied. For this reason I recommend the coloured version.

Why use masking fluid at all? Well let me explain, it allows you to paint over an area of your picture without letting the paint get on that area. Let's say you want to paint a background for a painting with flowers. First draw the outline of the flowers and then paint them with masking fluid. When the masking fluid is dry, paint your background and let it dry. Then rub off the masking fluid and you are then left with a white outline of the flowers. Now you can paint the flowers whatever colour you want. That's all there is to it.

Masking fluid is applied using a brush and I recommend you obtain a small cheap brush so you don't damage your good **Simply Painting** brushes.

If you don't have a cheap brush you can use your small **Simply Painting** Round Brush. However it is important to wash the brush out every twenty seconds or so, to stop the masking fluid sticking to the brush. If the masking fluid does harden on the brush, you can clean it with white spirits.

A word of warning, Murphy's Law states 'if anything can go wrong it will'. Masking fluid is difficult to remove from your clothes, it is therefore the most likely thing to spill. Remember Murphy's Law and be careful, as soon as you have finished using the masking fluid, replace the cap on the bottle and clean your brush in the water.

Also make sure the masking fluid is thoroughly dry before you paint over it because if it's not your brushes will stick to it.

Let me show you how it works.

1.   Draw the outline of the flowers and paint them with masking fluid.
2.   Then let it dry then paint the background ignoring the flowers.

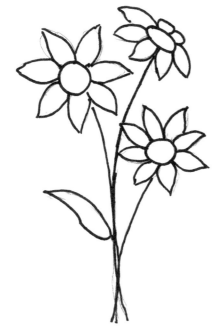

Fig. 1

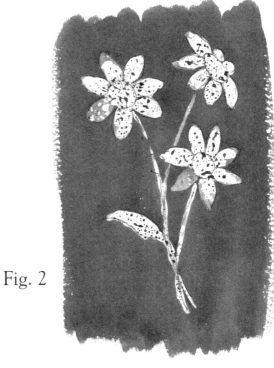

Fig. 2

3.   When the background is dry, rub off the masking fluid.
4.   Now paint the centres of the flowers and the stems.

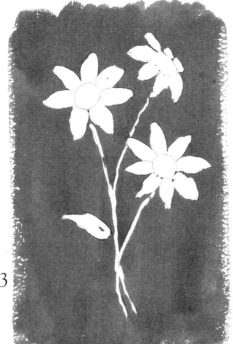

Fig. 3

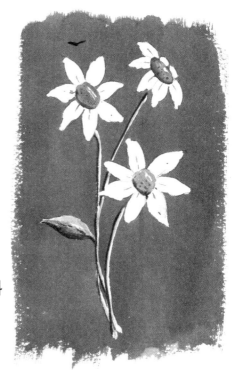

Fig. 4

Hairdryer

This is what I call my **Simply Painting** secret weapon. The reason I say this is that you can dry the painting faster and therefore control the paint better. If you have a hairdryer I do advise you to use it, however, just like the easel, a hairdryer is not an essential item of equipment.

This of course only applies when you are painting indoors, I don't think they make leads long enough for outdoor painting and it might also be a little dangerous. Hairdryers are only for use by artists over the age of sixteen.

Some Other Materials

- You will need a large container to hold the water. The larger the container the better, as the water will stay clean for a longer period. Try to find one which is not easily knocked over.

- While I have kept drawing to a minimum in these **Simply Painting** lessons, you will need a pencil for guidelines. A medium grade HB pencil is best for drawing light lines without damaging the paper.

- To attach your watercolour paper to the board you will need adhesive tape. I use masking tape which is easily obtained in a hardware store.

- An eraser is useful for rubbing out pencil lines. However be careful as an eraser can leave marks on the watercolour paper which damage it.

- You need a ruler to draw straight lines. As some of the lessons are painted on paper 14" (35cm) wide try to obtain one at least 20" (50cm) long.

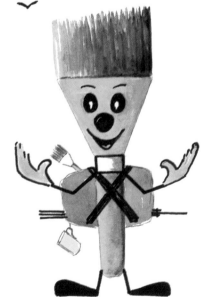

- Last, but by no means least, you need a cloth. We use the cloth for drying our brushes so it should be made of an absorbent material. I use a wad made by placing several household pads one on top of the other. These pads have a spongy texture and are ideal for drying the brushes.

2: How Does Have Some More Fun Work?

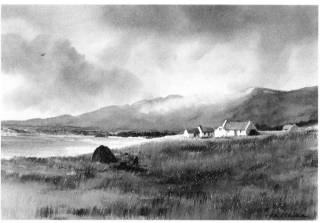

Well as I said before, someone has to show you how to start and it has to be simple. When I started to teach I found the one thing all beginners, and even some amateur painters, had in common was a very disorganised approach to their work. The same applied to me when I started to paint. I was unsure where to start and when I did, I was jumping about the paper like a bucket of frogs.

I was determined to devise a system which students found easy to use and remember. The answer was to break every picture into four distinct parts. Once they did this their painting improved in leaps and bounds.

However, as students left the class and may not have painted again for weeks or months, they seemed to forget what they were shown. So I racked my brain and found what I wanted in a simple unforgettable sentence, '**Have Some More Fun**'. The first letter of each of the four words represents how to paint a picture.

Have	=	H	=	Horizon
Some	=	S	=	Sky
More	=	M	=	Middleground
Fun	=	F	=	Foreground

In the following pictures you can see how this method works.

Have - Horizon

First, using your ruler, draw the horizon line straight across the board.

Some - Sky

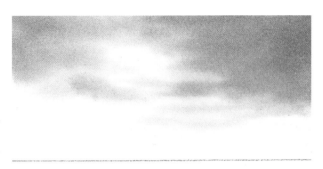

Then, starting at the top of your picture and keeping above the horizon line, paint the sky.

More - Middleground

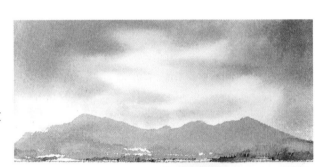

Next, just above the horizon line, paint a letter 'M' to represent the mountains.

Fun - Foreground

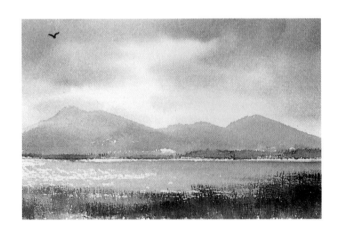

Lastly paint the foreground.

Have Some More Fun is the unique technique behind the **Simply Painting** concept and the method I use to paint all my pictures.

If you use this chapter as your guiding light you will begin to realise how simple and enjoyable painting is and you too will be able to **Have Some More Fun**.

3: Brush Strokes

The reason you need only two *Simply Painting* brushes to start painting watercolours is that they can perform many different tasks. Also you won't be confused by too much equipment, not to mention the cost of purchasing many different brushes.

As the saying goes, 'a good workman knows and minds his tools'. Before you start to paint, let me show you how to use the brushes.

The *Simply Painting* **Large Brush** is in fact three brushes in one.

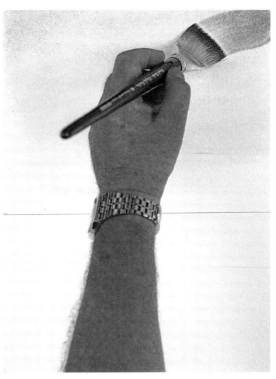

First it is a wash brush used for covering large areas quickly.

This is done using broad strokes and is essential for painting skies. I will go so far as to say it is impossible to paint wet onto wet watercolour skies without using a large wash brush.

Secondly, by using the tip it can paint narrow strokes.

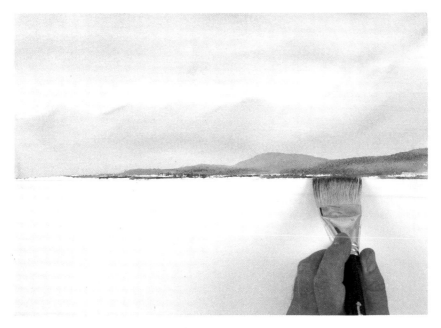

Last, but by no means least, you can use the corner to dab on the paint. This is great for foliage, bushes, and trees etc.

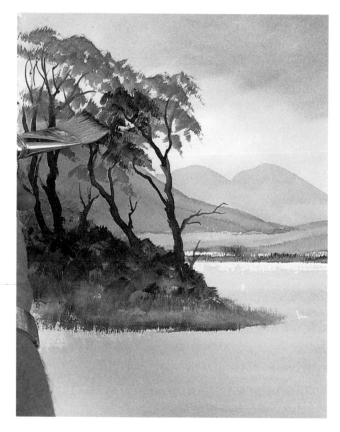

The small **Simply Painting Round Brush** is made of nylon and is ideal for painting detail.

I tell my students to use it like they would a pen or pencil.

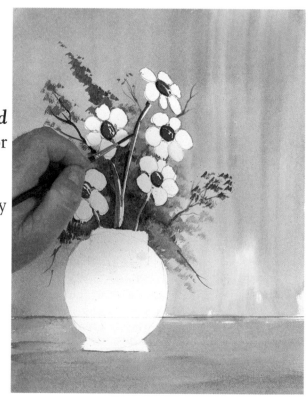

4: Using Water with the Large Brush

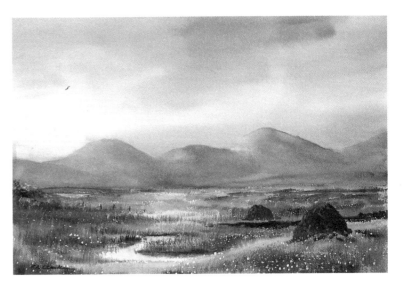

As the name suggests, with watercolour painting you use water, but how much and how do you control it? In my art classes these are the most often asked questions and rightly so.

The **Simply Painting** Large Brush can, because of its size, hold a lot of water and we need to control the amount of water on the large brush. One way to let your picture get out of control is to use too much water.

Question: How do you control the water?

Answer: With the cloth.

For the purposes of simplicity let's break the hair of the large brush into two parts, the tip and the body. The tip is the top half inch (12mm) of the hair and body is the rest of the hair.

Tip = Top .5 inch (12mm) of the hair

Body = The rest of the hair

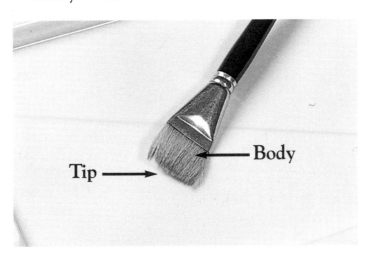

When you want to control the amount of water in your large brush this is what you do:

1. Dip your brush into the water.

2. Using your cloth, dry the body of the brush by resting it on the cloth.

DO NOT DRY THE TIP

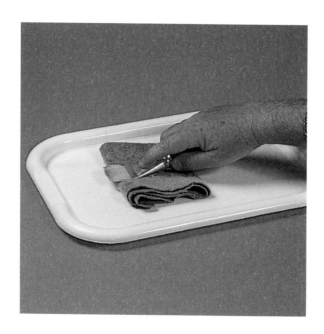

This allows the tip to remain wet, and ensures that there is not too much water in the body of the brush.

3. Now dip the brush into the paint and apply it to the paper.

This process is repeated every time you want to apply paint to your picture. With a little practice, you will get to know just how much water you need in the large brush.

When wetting the paper without any paint on your large brush there is no need to dry the body with the cloth. Small brushes do not retain much water so there is little need to use this technique with them.

5: The Two Minute Sky

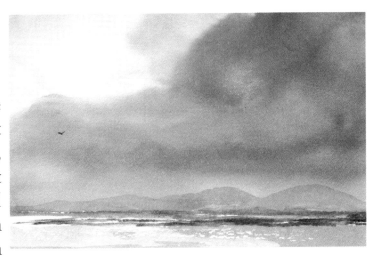

Before you start to paint let me say that the sky is the most important part of any painting, because if the sky is right the rest of your painting will be right. I believe if you were to take a piece of paper everyday for a week and paint a sky, you'd be a watercolorist, because it is a key part of the picture.

However you've only got two minutes to paint the sky, no longer. After two minutes, the paper tends to dry and it's hard to get the pigment onto the paper.

When painting skies with watercolours using the **Have Some More Fun** system, I use a wet into wet method which means wetting the watercolour paper first and then painting the sky while the paper is still wet.

This method has the effect of turning the paper into blotting paper thus allowing the paint to spread and gives a soft effect to the sky.

However the sky must be completed before the paper starts to dry, otherwise you will get hard edges and marks in your sky. This is what I mean when I say the two minute sky!

NOW THE FUN BEGINS!

Mountain Scene

FOR THIS LESSON YOU WILL NEED THE FOLLOWING MATERIALS

1.5" (38MM) WINSOR & NEWTON *Simply Painting* LARGE BRUSH

WINSOR & NEWTON *Simply Painting* SMALL BRUSH

1 SHEET OF 140 LBS (300 GSM) WATERCOLOUR PAPER 10" x 14" (25 X 35 CMS)

20" x 16" (50 X 40 CMS) BOARD

CONTAINER OF WATER, PENCIL, CLOTH, RULER, ADHESIVE TAPE.

A HAIRDRYER, IF YOU HAVE ONE.

WATERCOLOUR PAINTS

RAW SIENNA • BURNT UMBER • COBALT BLUE HUE

6: Mountain Scene

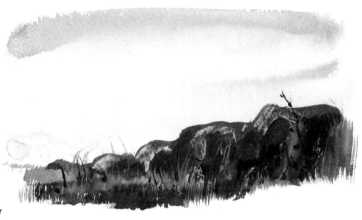

Painting is about enjoying yourself and having fun. If you have never painted before, don't worry, there is no mistake you can make in watercolour painting that I haven't already made, so if you follow me, you will surprise yourself. This mountain scene is on the road to Clifden in the West of Ireland, but it could be anywhere. When you have completed this lesson you can then paint a mountain scene from your own area.

First of all, gather the materials together and look at the finished picture, then read the lesson in full <u>before</u> you start to paint.

Step 1: Have - Horizon

Let's begin. This picture is in landscape (longwise) so, using the tape, attach a sheet of paper by three corners to the board making sure there is a long side at the bottom.

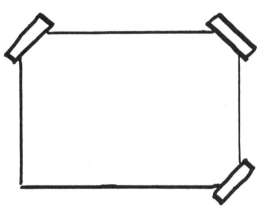

Next draw the horizon line using your ruler and pencil, about one-third of the way up the page.

23

Step 2: Some - Sky

For the this lesson, we need three colours but for now just put out some Raw Sienna and Cobalt Blue Hue onto the side of your palette. To paint the sky let's wet the paper with a light wash of Raw Sienna using the large brush.

Take some Raw Sienna into the centre of your palette, not too much. Then starting from the top of the paper, paint as if you are painting a door. Make broad horizontal brush strokes back and forward across the paper.

Continue down until you come to within one inch from the horizon line. This will leave a pale light brown tint on the paper. Don't use too much paint in the mixture.

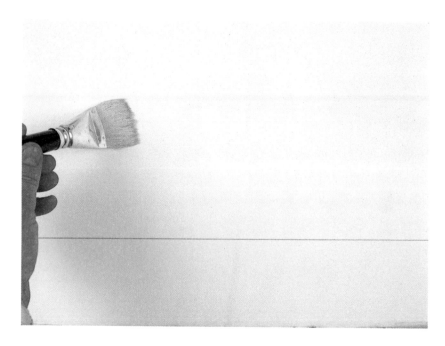

Now back to your palette while the paper is still damp and using Cobalt Blue Hue, paint in some blue sky.

Start once again at the top of the paper and make sure that you **complete the sky within the two minutes allowed.**

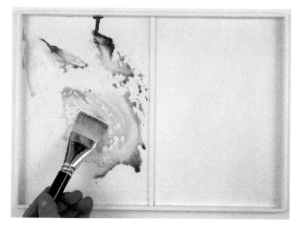

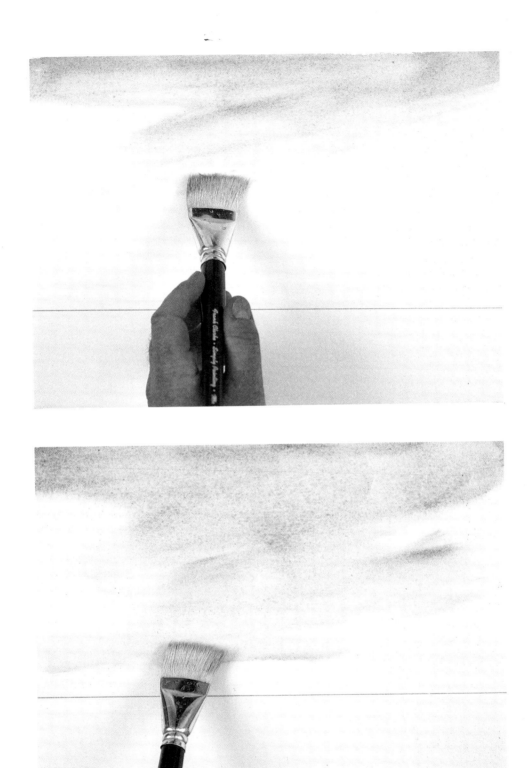

When you have completed the sky, let the paper dry. When you are painting with watercolours it is important to remember to let your picture dry before painting over it again.

If you continue painting over a wet sky you will make a mess of your picture. You can use a hairdryer if you have one but if you don't, then wait until the sky is completely dry before continuing. This will take about five minutes

Tip: Keep looking at the finished picture. After all, it's what you are painting and remember if you are not happy with your sky, you can turn the paper over and start again. I often do this myself.

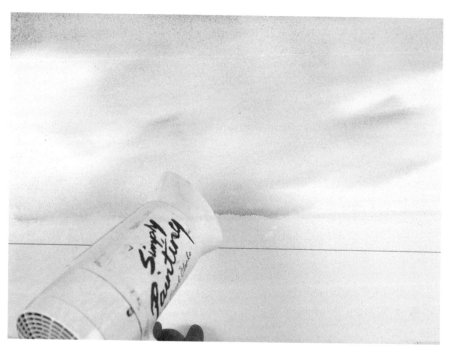

Step 3: More - Middleground

Next let's paint the mountains. These mountains are part of the beautiful Twelve Pins in Connemara. I know them so well I could paint them from memory and often do.

If you look at the finished picture you will see that the mountains are far away and are very faint. The further away the mountains are the lighter they become.

So let's paint the distant mountains first using the large brush with a mixture of Raw Sienna and Cobalt Blue Hue, 25% Raw Sienna and 75% Cobalt Blue Hue.

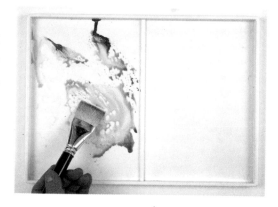

Start on the right hand side and paint a large letter M across the page, then fill it in.

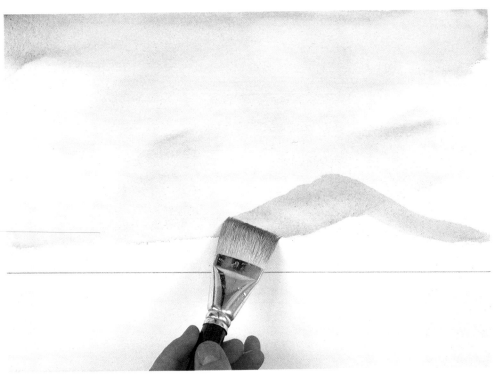

The mountains on the left hand side are darker, so let's paint them darker by adding more Cobalt Blue Hue to the mixture.

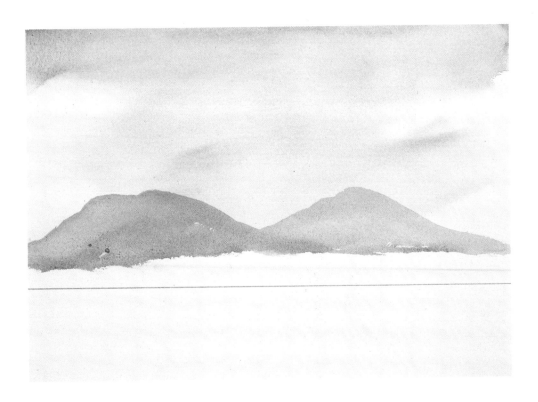

That completes the mountain range, so once again let your picture dry.

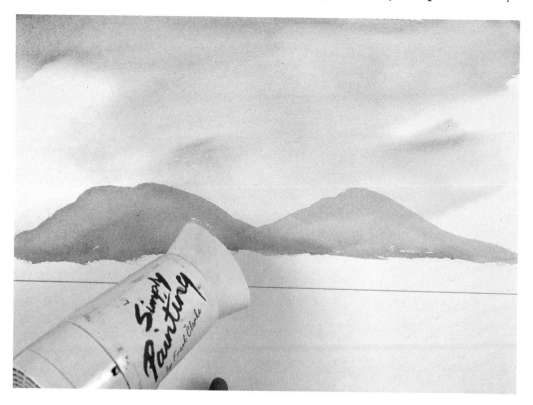

Put out some Burnt Umber on the edge of the palette. Now let's paint the middleground which stretches between the mountains and the riverbank.

For this we need green which in this case is made by mixing mostly Raw Sienna and a tiny amount of Cobalt Blue Hue.

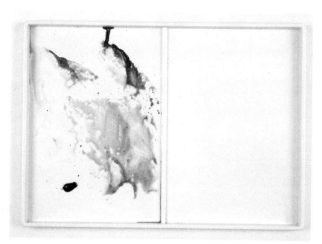

Using the large brush, mix some Raw Sienna with a small amount of Cobalt Blue on the palette.

Tip: Mix your paints on the palette, not on the paper, it will avoid MUD, a colour well known to all beginners.

Paint the land below the mountains being careful to keep above the horizon line. Again look at the finished picture before you start.

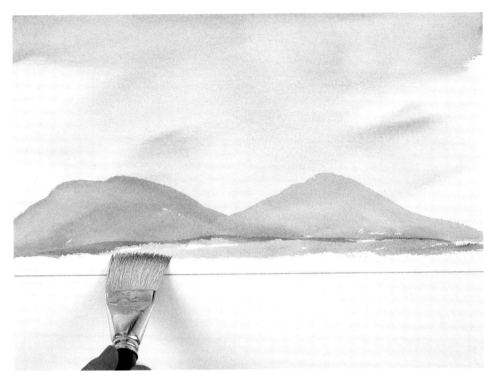

Vary the colours by adding a little more Cobalt Blue Hue. Don't fill it in completely, leave some white bits here and there. This creates texture in the picture.

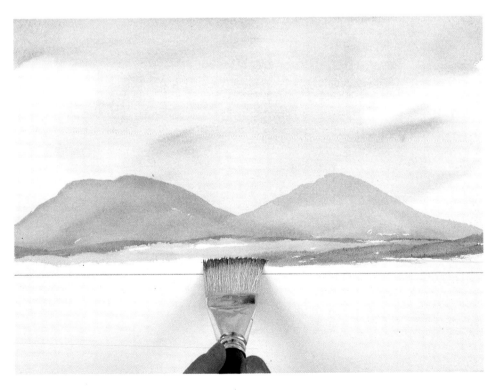

Usually when you have a lake, you have a muddy bank, so let's darken across the horizon line to represent this bank. Don't go below the horizon line.

To do this use the large brush and mix equal amounts of Burnt Umber and Raw Sienna.

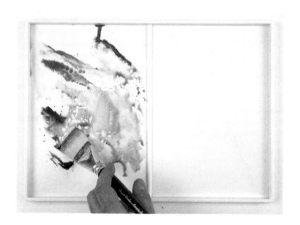

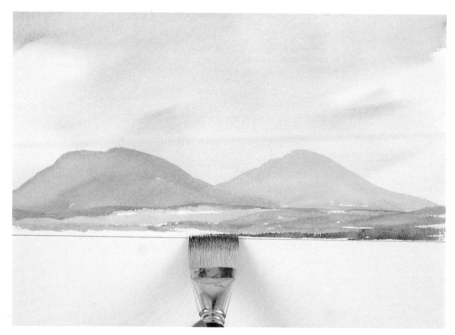

Dab it right on the horizon line and this will give the impression of a distant riverbank.

If you want to make it darker add more Burnt Umber, remember it's your riverbank.

When you have completed this dry your picture.

Use your hairdryer or wait until it is dry before starting to paint the water.

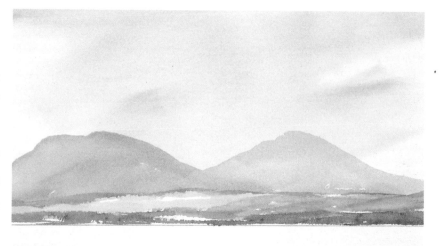

Step 4: Fun - Foreground

Now we are ready to paint the lake. Take the large brush from the water and dry it on the cloth. Using Cobalt Blue Hue with broad horizontal strokes, paint the water.

Tip: Mix enough paint before you start painting the water.

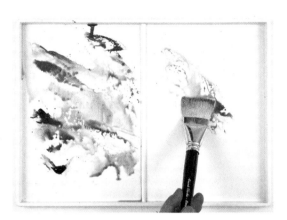

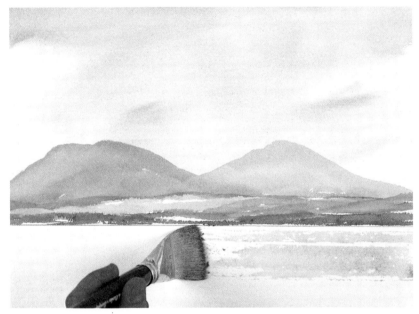

Once you start, don't stop, go right across continuing to the bottom of the paper.

It may take four or five strokes and in some cases you may have to go over the water again. If you do just remember to complete the stroke right across the paper.

When you are finished, dry it.

If you find that the water isn't dark enough wait until it has dried and go over it again with more paint.

This process is known as laying washes.

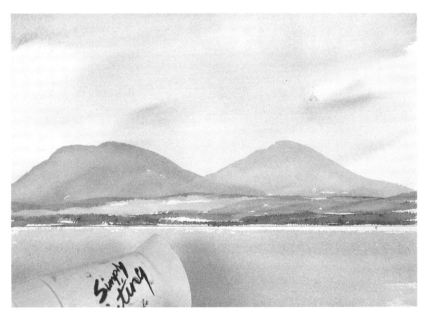

Lastly, we come to the reeds or rushes, which we paint using Burnt Umber only.

Dry the large brush on the cloth and pick up some Burnt Umber.

Paint the reeds right across the bottom of the picture. Use broad downward strokes.

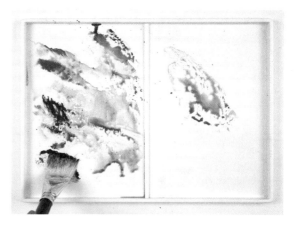

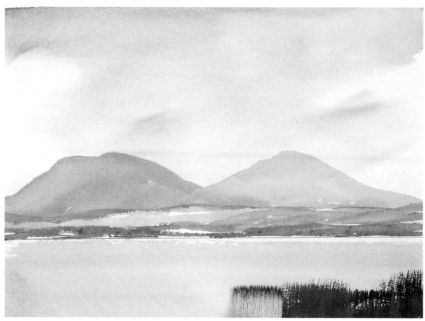

You can vary the colour as you are painting by adding a little water, but be careful don't use too much water. Keep the brush fairly dry.

When you are finished let it dry.

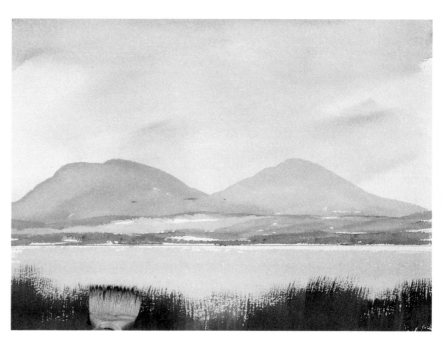

32

When that's completed, let's add a little life to the scene by painting some birds. How do you draw a bird? You take the letter V and flatten it. I always put a little bird in the corner, it has become my trade mark.

So using a pen or brush, draw or paint some flat letter Vs for the birds. Make both wings the same size.

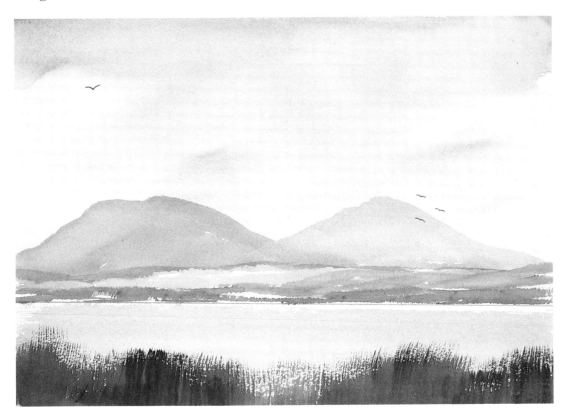

Well done, you have completed your picture.

Now Sign it.

Congratulations.

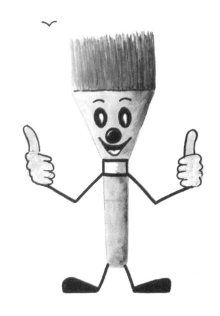

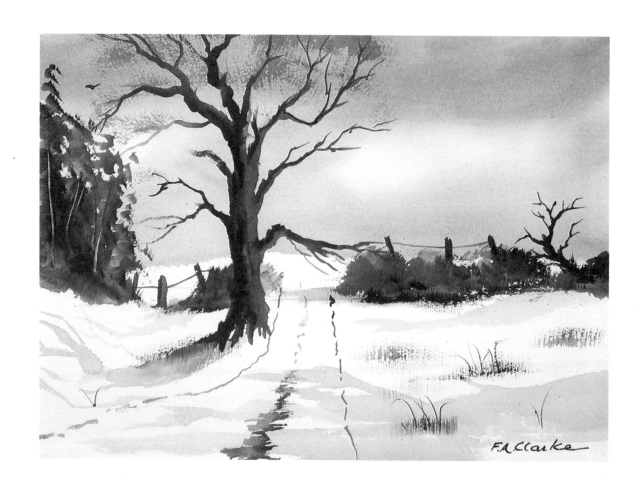

SNOW SCENE

FOR THIS LESSON YOU WILL NEED THE FOLLOWING MATERIALS

1.5" (38MM) WINSOR & NEWTON *Simply Painting* LARGE BRUSH

WINSOR & NEWTON *Simply Painting* SMALL BRUSH

1 SHEET OF 140 LB (300 GSM) WATERCOLOUR PAPER 10" x 14" (25 X 35 CMS)

20" x 16" (50 X 40 CMS) BOARD

CONTAINER OF WATER, PENCIL, CLOTH, RULER, ADHESIVE TAPE.

A HAIRDRYER, IF YOU HAVE ONE.

WATERCOLOUR PAINTS

RAW SIENNA • ALIZARIN CRIMSON • COBALT BLUE HUE

• BURNT UMBER

7: Snow Scene

I always enjoy painting snow scenes, they make great presents and of course, being a mean artist, I don't have to use much paint because I can use the paper as my white paint.

Step 1: Have -Horizon

First affix your sheet of paper by three corners to the board with the tape. Put two at the top and one at the bottom. We are painting this in landscape, so make sure one of the long sides is at the bottom.

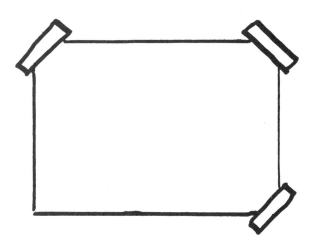

Take your ruler and pencil and draw the horizon line, just under half way up the paper.

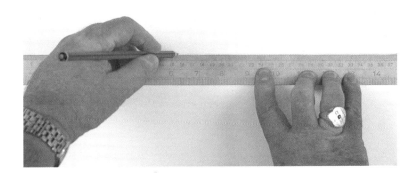

Step 2: Some - Sky

The colours we going to use for the sky are Raw Sienna, Cobalt Blue Hue, and Alizarin Crimson, so squeeze some of each onto the side of your palette, keeping them well apart.

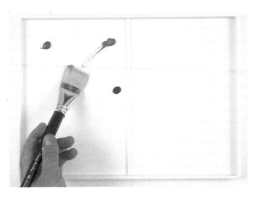

Dip the large brush into the water and dry it on the cloth. Take some Raw Sienna to the centre of the palette and make an inky mixture with the Raw Sienna and water.

Make sure that the colour is a light mixture, that is, not too much paint. Now starting from the top of the paper, paint down to within an inch of the horizon line. Remember you have only two minutes to paint the sky.

Use broad horizontal brush strokes back and forward to give an even coat of paint on the paper. This will leave a pale light brown tint on the paper.

Now, while the paint and the paper is still wet, take some Cobalt Blue Hue and Alizarin Crimson, equal amounts of each, and make a purple mixture on the palette.

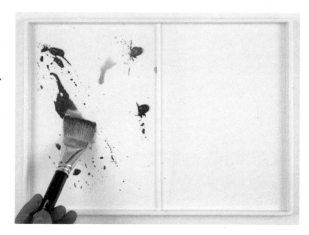

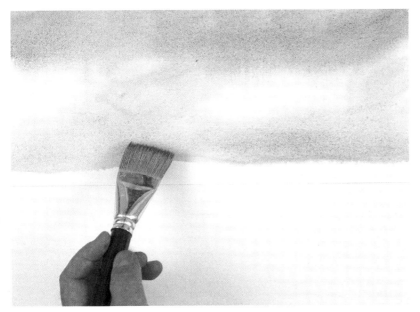

Starting from the top of the picture, paint in the sky, leaving some white areas to represent clouds.

That completes the sky, so now dry it. Use a hairdryer if you have one, if not, just wait until the sky is dry before continuing. Relax and enjoy your hobby, there is no hurry at this stage. Clean your large brush in the water and then have a cup of coffee if you wish.

Step 3: More - Middleground

Now starting on the right hand side of the picture, let's paint the bushes using the large brush with a mixture of Raw Sienna only, paint the hedge above the horizon line, on the right hand side of the picture. Be careful that you don't go too far across the page, look at the finished painting.

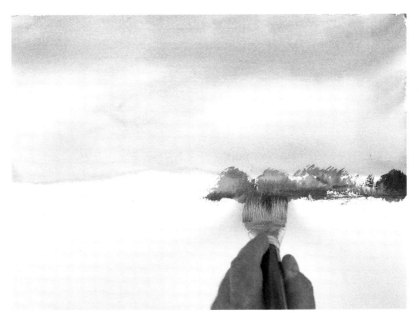

Now put out some Burnt Umber onto the side of your palette and add some darker colour to the bushes using Burnt Umber only. To give the bushes a nice shape use the corner of the large brush. When you are finished, clean your large brush in the water.

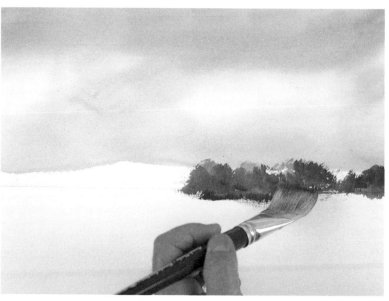

Step 4: Fun - Foreground

Now let's paint the roadway. First we draw it with the small brush using some Raw Sienna and a tiny bit of Burnt Umber. Look at the finished picture and you will notice that the right side of the roadway runs almost straight down to the bottom of the paper, while the left hand side runs in a semi-circle out to the edge of the paper. This will give the impression that the road is wider at the bottom of the picture. Outline the road with a broken line.

Having done that, using the small brush with Raw Sienna, paint the centre of the roadway. This is the higher ground in the centre of the road where the snow has melted. As it goes up towards the horizon line, it gets narrower. This gives the impression of distance.

Now that we have the road defined we can paint the bushes on the left hand side. Look at the finished picture and using Raw Sienna only with the corner of the large brush, create a dip in the ground by painting below the horizon line and back above the horizon line again.

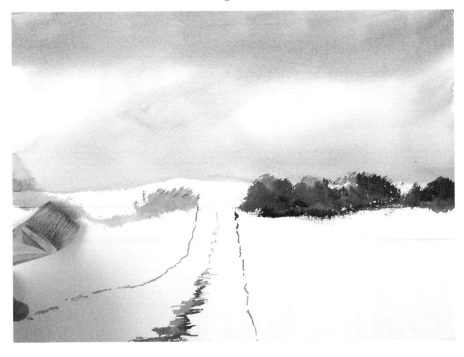

Darken the hedge on the left hand side with Burnt Umber in the same way you did with the hedges on the right hand side.

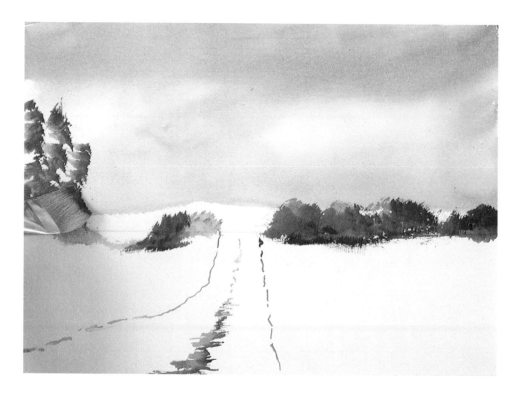

Then paint the trees on the left hand side with equal amounts of Raw Sienna and Burnt Umber. Use the corner of the large brush to dab the paint on.

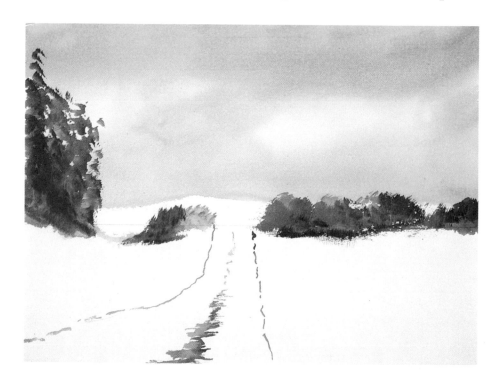

With your fingernail, scrape out some tree trunks on the trees on the left hand side. Don't do too many.

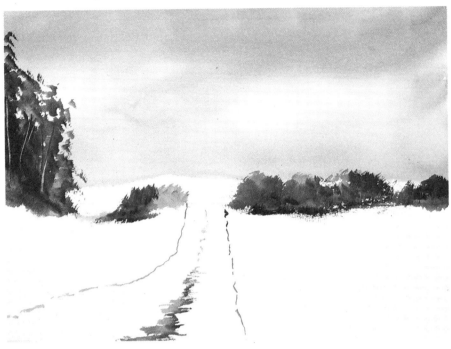

Next we have to paint the large tree which is the main point of interest in this painting.

With the small brush and using Raw Sienna, start by painting the skeleton of the tree from the ground up. That's the way trees grow - from the ground up.

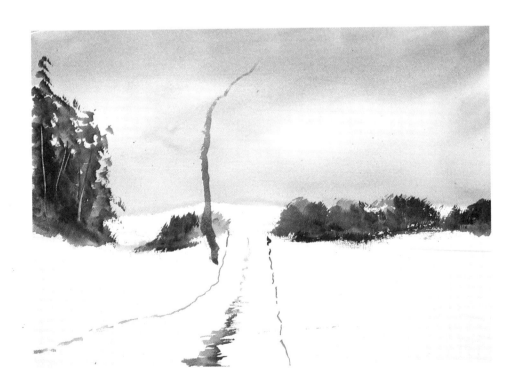

You will notice that the base of the tree is lower on the left hand side than it is on the right hand side. This is because the tree is growing on a slope. Paint it all in Raw Sienna first.

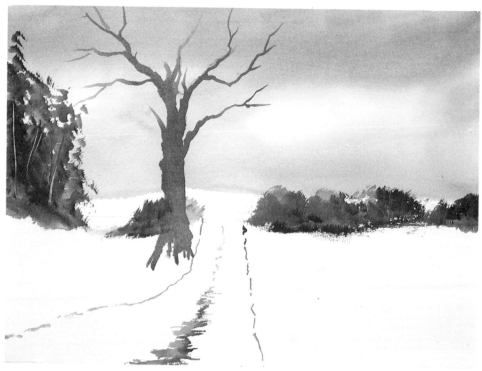

Now paint a little Burnt Umber on the left hand side of the tree to give it some shadows. Again drag your brush from the ground up.

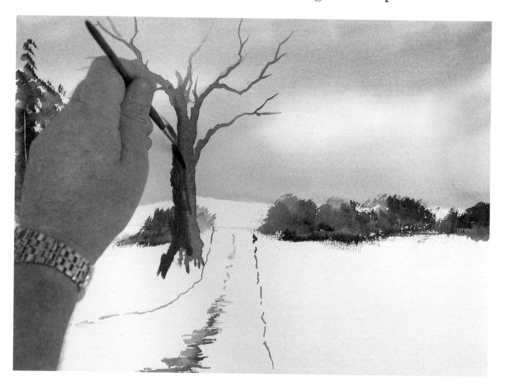

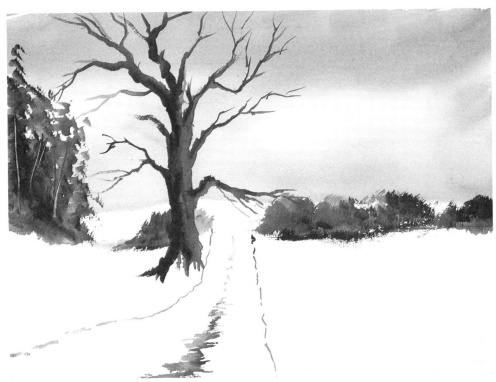

Having completed the skeleton of the tree, we now paint the fences on the right and left of the roadway. Use the small brush with Burnt Umber only and begin by painting the posts. These are old posts so don't paint them too straight. When you are finished, paint the wire that joins the posts. Let it sag a little to make the fence look old.

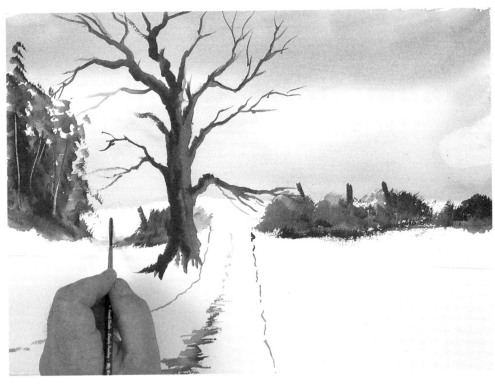

There is no need to paint snow as we can use the white paper for the snow, so the next thing we have to paint are the shadows on the ground.

These shadows are created using the same colour as the sky, which in this case was equal amounts of Cobalt Blue Hue and Alizarin Crimson.

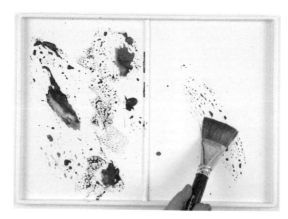

So mix up some Cobalt Blue Hue and Alizarin Crimson, exactly the same as the colour you mixed for the sky but this time don't make it too strong -use a little more water.

Then, starting just underneath the fence, paint in some shadows on the left and right of the picture.

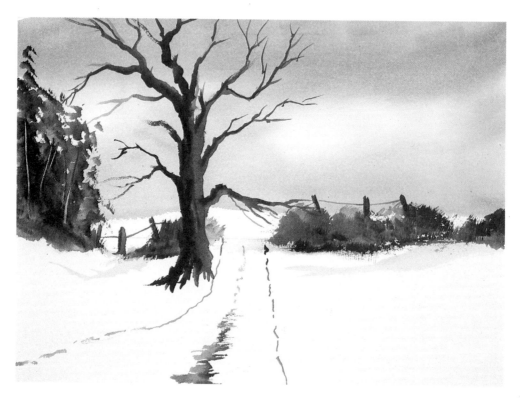

Now look carefully at the finished picture. There's a valley behind and to the left of the tree, so naturally the shadow of the tree must run down into the valley and up again.

To paint this valley start below the base of the tree and draw your large brush down and then up again towards the bushes on the left.

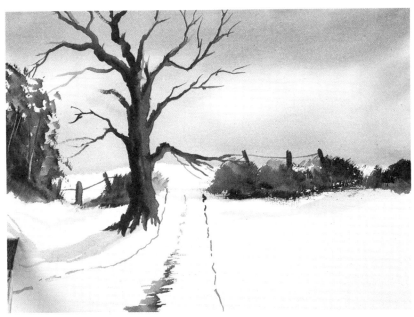

There is another tree on the right hand side, it's just out of the picture so we can't see it. Its shadow runs along the bottom of the picture and over the roadway. So using the large brush paint this shadow using the same colour you used for the other ones. Notice how it too bends down on the right of the roadway to show that there is a dip there too.

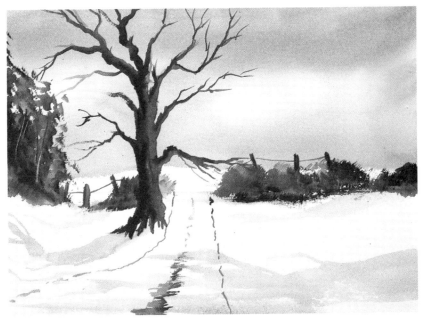

Now lastly, as the snow is beginning to melt, we need to paint the little bits of grass which have sprung up through the snow.

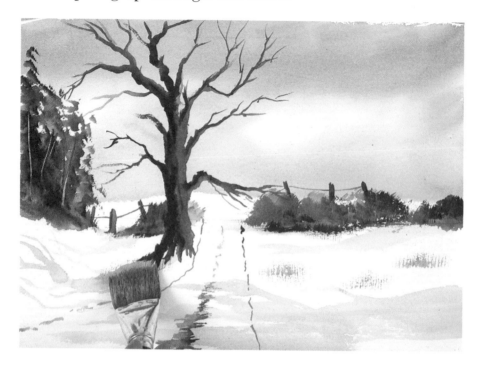

Using Raw Sienna on your large brush create some grass using downward strokes with the large brush.

Darken the colour by adding a little Burnt Umber to it and paint this darker colour on the grass here and there.

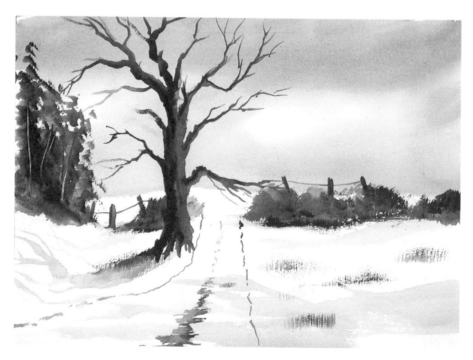

That just about completes the foreground. We have one or two things left to do and the first is to put twigs on the trees. It's a winter scene, so there are only twigs not leaves on the trees.

So with the large brush extremely dry, and using a mixture of 2/3 Raw Sienna and 1/3 Burnt Umber, make downward strokes with the

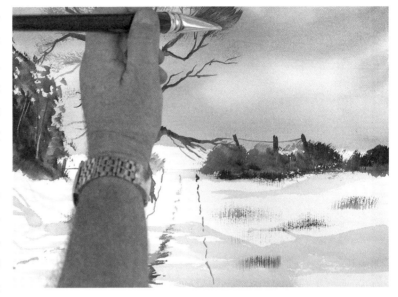

corner of the brush to denote some twigs at the top of the tree. Don't overdo this.

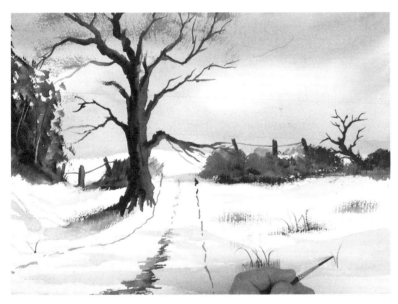

With the small brush paint a little tree on the right hand side above the fence. Do this exactly as you painted the large tree except this time use Burnt Umber only.

While you're at it, put some flecks of tall grass coming up through the snow with the Burnt Umber.

And last but by no means least, I am going to paint my bird up in the top left hand corner. You however can paint him anywhere you wish. That completes our snow scene.

Finally, sign it.

Well done.

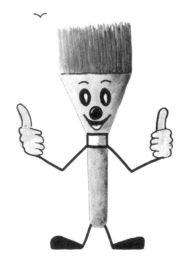

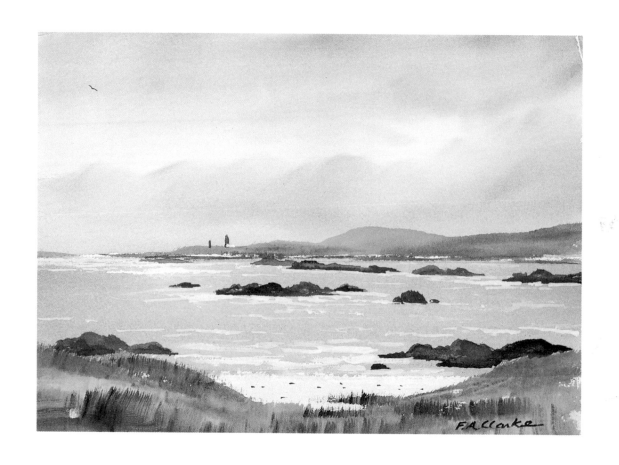

LIGHTHOUSE AT SLYNE HEAD

FOR THIS LESSON YOU WILL NEED THE FOLLOWING MATERIALS

1.5" (38MM) WINSOR & NEWTON *Simply Painting* LARGE BRUSH

WINSOR & NEWTON *Simply Painting* SMALL BRUSH

1 SHEET OF 140 LB (300 GSM) WATERCOLOUR PAPER 10" x 14" (25 X 35 CMS)

20" x 16" (50 X 40 CMS) BOARD

CONTAINER OF WATER, PENCIL, CLOTH, RULER, ADHESIVE TAPE.

A HAIRDRYER, IF YOU HAVE ONE.

WATERCOLOUR PAINTS

RAW SIENNA • LIGHT RED • COBALT BLUE HUE

LEMON YELLOW HUE • BURNT UMBER • DESIGNER'S WHITE GOUACHE

8: *Lighthouse at Slyne Head*

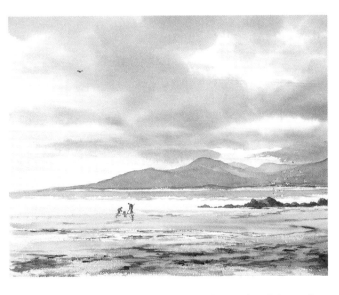

This is a view looking across Ballyconneely Bay towards Slyne Head lighthouse in County Galway. The lighthouse was originally built in 1850 and was one of the last lighthouses in Ireland to be manned, but has recently been made automatic.

This beautiful scene is close to my studio. The lighthouse is often hidden by fog but on this occasion I had a clear view for miles out to sea.

Step 1: Have - Horizon

This picture is painted in landscape, so using the tape, attach your paper to the board on three sides with one of the long sides at the bottom.

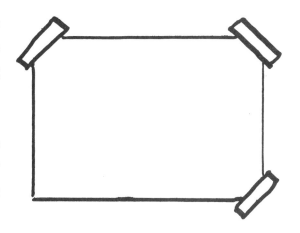

The horizon line is just under half way up the paper, so using your pencil and a ruler draw the horizon line about 6" from the bottom of the paper.

Step2: Some - Sky

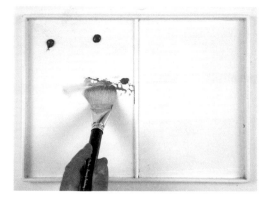

Now put out some Raw Sienna, Cobalt Blue Hue and Light Red on your palette.

Take some Raw Sienna and starting from the top, paint down to within a quarter of an inch of the horizon line. Make sure that the paint is a light mixture. Use very little Raw Sienna with the water, we just want to tint the paper.

Tip: Remember the two minute rule when painting the sky.

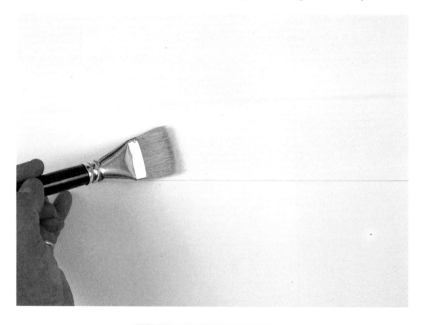

Now, while the paper is still wet, take some Cobalt Blue Hue and starting from the top of the picture, paint the sky, leaving some unpainted areas to represent clouds.

While the sky is still wet, take 25% Light Red and 75% Cobalt Blue Hue, and paint a darker strip along the bottom of the horizon line.

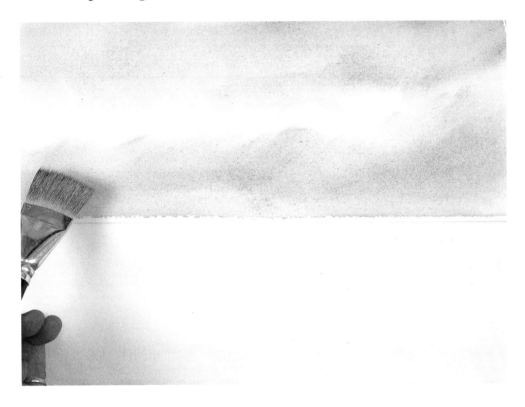

Now let it dry or if you have a hairdryer use it. That completes the sky.

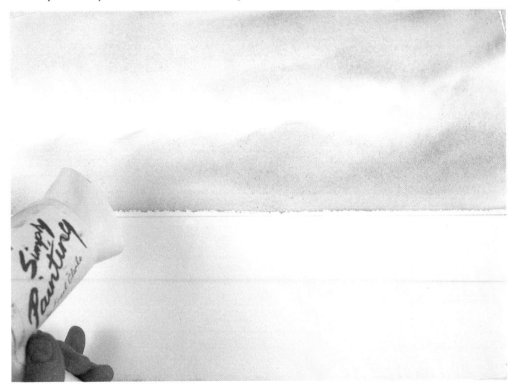

Step 3: More - Middleground

Before you start to paint the middleground add some Lemon Yellow Hue and Burnt Umber to the palette. Now you should have five colours around the edge of your palette.

The middleground is mainly a green colour and this is made with a mixture of Lemon Yellow Hue, Raw Sienna and a small amount of Cobalt Blue Hue.

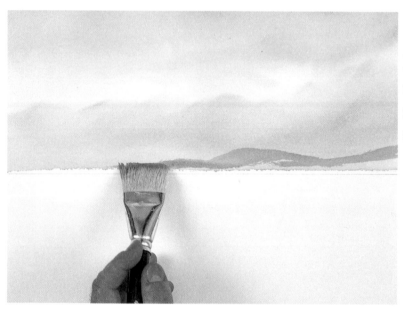

Paint the faraway coastline using this mixture with narrow horizontal strokes of the large brush.

As you paint, vary the colour slightly by picking up different combinations of these paints from the palette.

In other words, add in some Raw Sienna or a little Cobalt Blue Hue to give an impression of different tones in the distance.

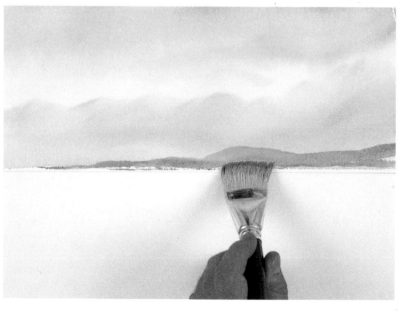

Finally with the large brush and Burnt Umber, paint the seashore in the distance along the horizon line. Leave some unpainted areas here and there for effect. Now dry the picture with your hairdryer or wait until it dries before painting the sea.

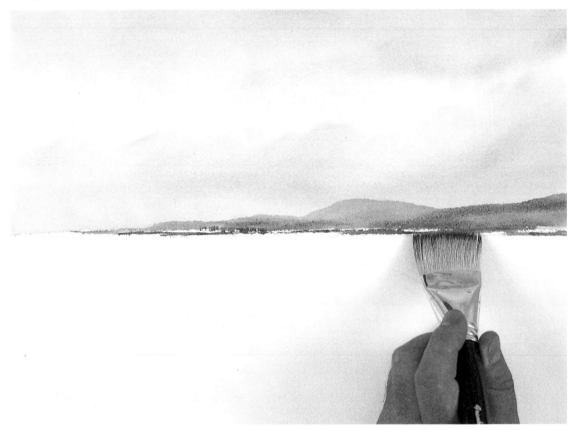

Step 4: Fun - Foreground

Now we come to the sea. We want the sea to look the same colour as the sky, so use the same colours for the sea that were used in the sky.

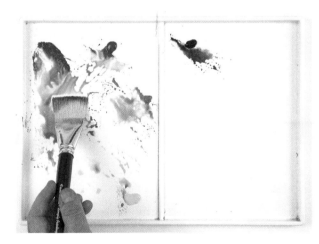

In this scene the sea is made up of Cobalt Blue Hue and a tiny bit of Light Red which are the same colours we used for the sky.

So with the large brush, mix some Cobalt Blue Hue and Light Red together.

Then put the brush on the right hand side of the paper and using broad horizontal strokes paint the sea. Once you start, don't stop, otherwise you will get marks across the sea that you don't want.

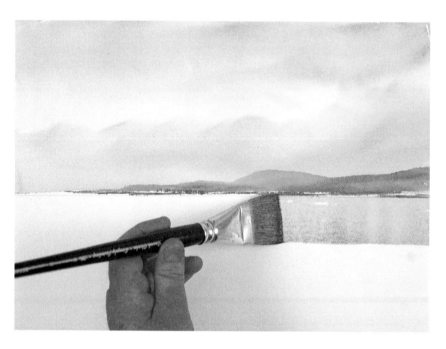

Keep repeating this stroke underneath until you reach about 2" from the bottom of the paper. Look at the finished picture.

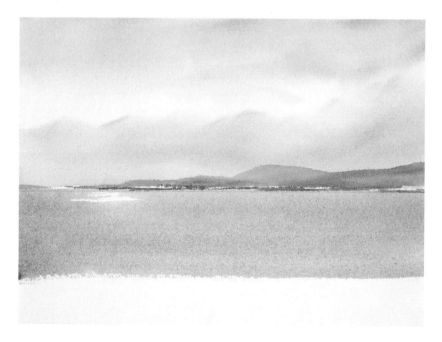

If the sea is not dark enough, dry it and then paint over it again. You will notice I left a little piece of white paper unpainted. This is known as a 'happy mistake', but don't try to make it happen.

Then dry the sea. Use your hairdryer, if you have one.

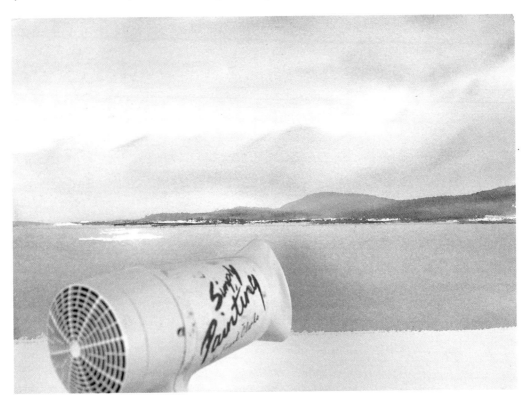

Tip: Don't put the hairdryer too near the paper or it will move the pigment on you. Keep the point of the hairdryer about 2" or 3" away when you are drying your picture.

When you've completed the water, look at the rocks in the sea. To paint them take your small brush, dip it into the water and dry it off. Use a mixture of Burnt Umber and a little Cobalt Blue Hue to paint the rocks.

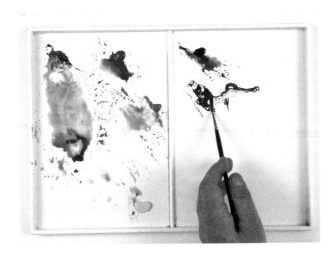

Start with the furthest ones which are a slightly lighter colour. To obtain this, use more water with the paint and progressively add more colour as you paint the rocks nearer to the shore.

Make sure that the bottom of each rock is parallel to the horizon line.

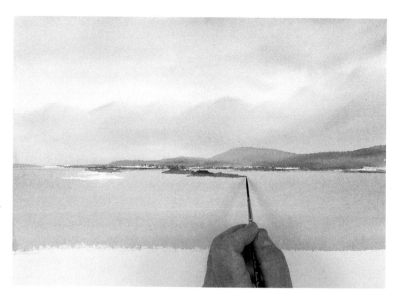

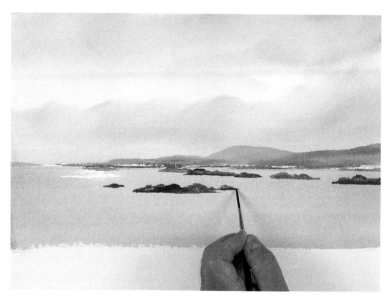

You can always darken the rocks later if you're not happy with them by adding some darker paint but remember to dry them first.

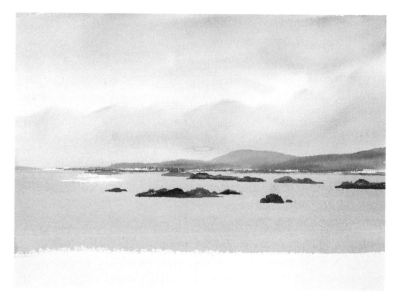

Now to complete the foreground let's paint the beach using Raw Sienna only, use the same mixture you used for the wash in the sky.

Paint the beach in the same way as you did the sea, using broad horizontal strokes.

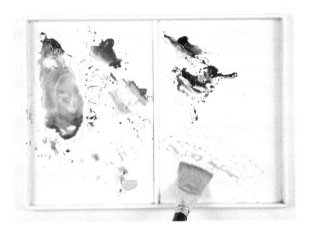

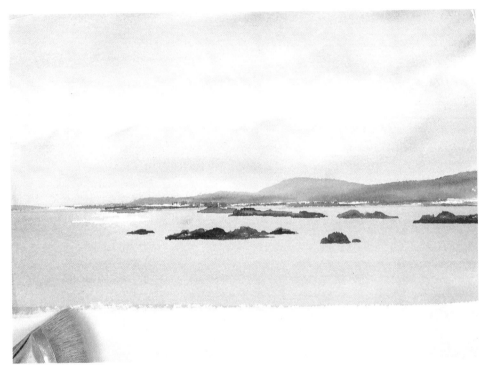

Wasn't that easy. Now let it dry.

Our next task is to paint the sand dunes and the grass bank in the foreground.

This is done with a mixture of Lemon Yellow Hue, Raw Sienna and Cobalt Blue Hue, using a little more Lemon Yellow Hue than the other two.

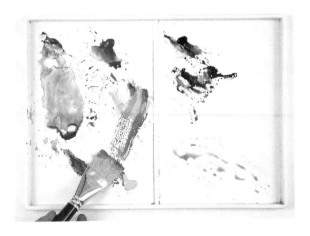

57

Use the large brush and paint right across the bottom of the picture leaving a dip in the centre so the beach will be seen between the sand dunes.

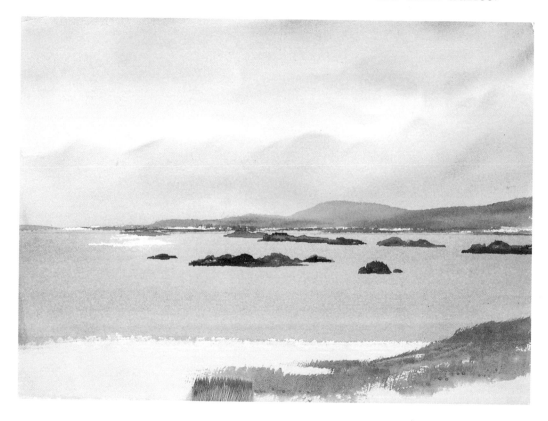

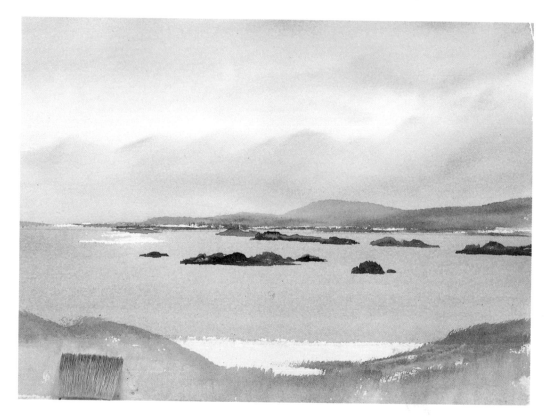

To paint the grass in the foreground, start on one side, whichever side you like, and with broad downward strokes of the large brush, paint some Burnt Umber while the sand dunes are still wet.

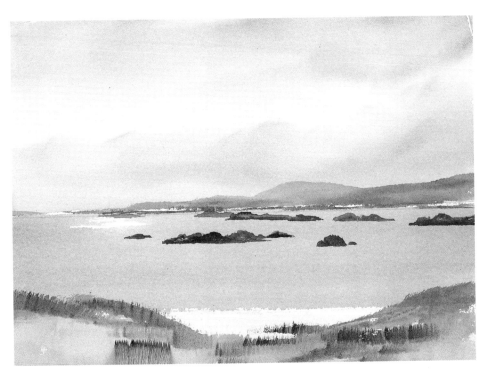

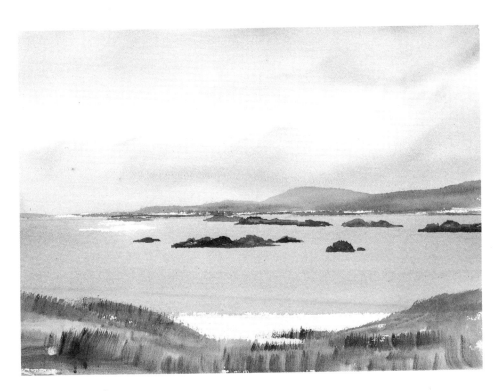

Now let the picture dry.

That completes the foreground, except for the rocks, which we paint with the small brush. This time we need Burnt Umber, Cobalt Blue Hue and a little Light Red. Make them a little darker than the ones in the distance.

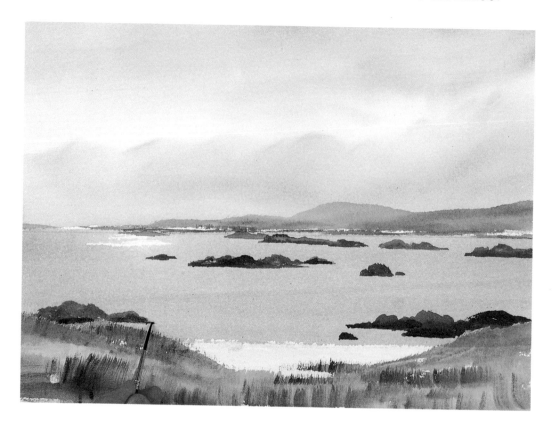

When you have completed the rocks in the foreground on the right and left, there are only a couple of things left to do.

We have to paint the lighthouse and of course, the waves in the sea. The sea looks very flat at the moment, so how could we change it?

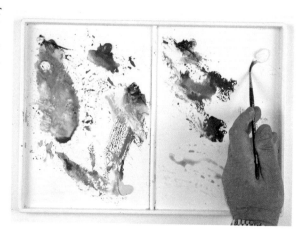

Well, we have our secret weapon which is called White Gouache, so squeeze some out onto the side of your palette.

Tip: If you can't get White Gouache, Chinese White will do.

60

Using the small brush, create a sunlit area on the left of the sea under the horizon line. Now you can see why, when I left some of the sea unpainted, I called it a 'happy mistake'.

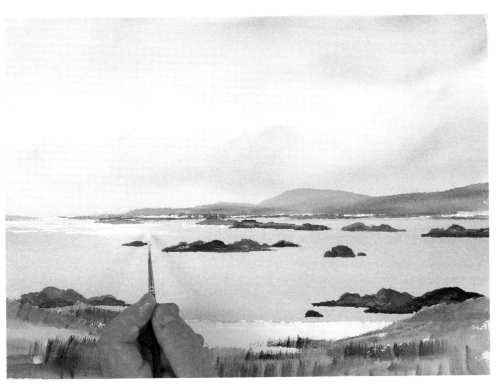

We also use the White Gouache to paint in the waves near the shore.

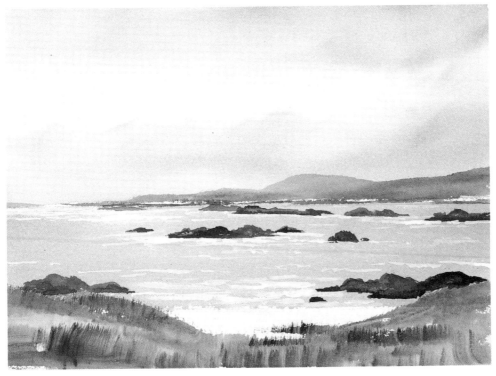

Now last but by no means least we are going to paint the twin lighthouses. The one on the left is abandoned, and the one on the right is in use. These are just two single downward strokes with the small brush. Use Light Red and a little Burnt Umber. Don't make them too big, they are not sky scrapers.

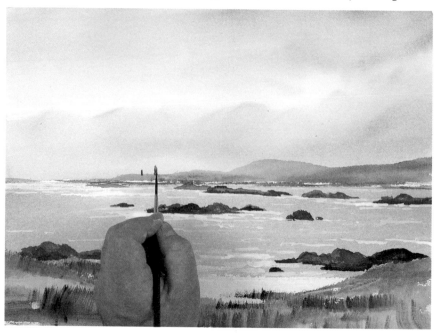

Let the picture dry before you go any further. Let's put in the living accommodation, which is the block of white on the right hand side. It is connected to the main lighthouse and is just barely visible. Paint it with a small dab of White Gouache, have a good look at the finished painting.

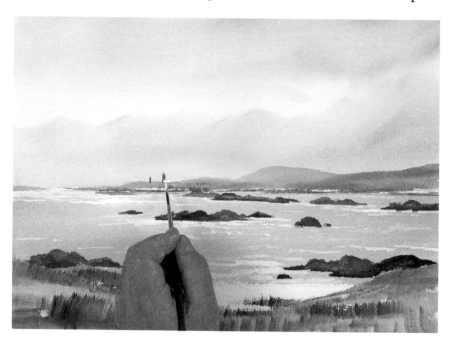

Paint some pebbles on the beach with the small brush.

They are just little dots of Burnt Umber.

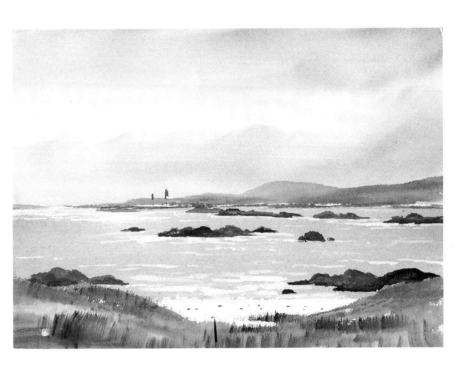

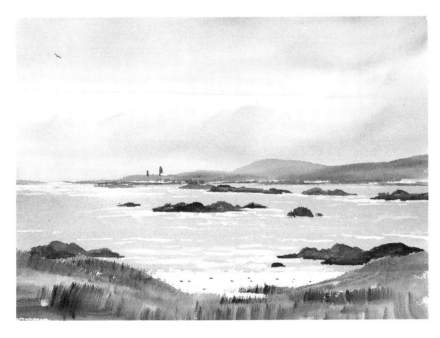

Lastly, you can put in some birds. I am just going to paint my friend in the left corner.

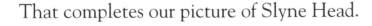

That completes our picture of Slyne Head.

Now sign it.

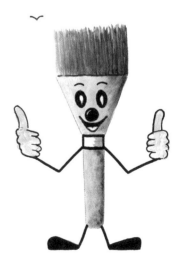

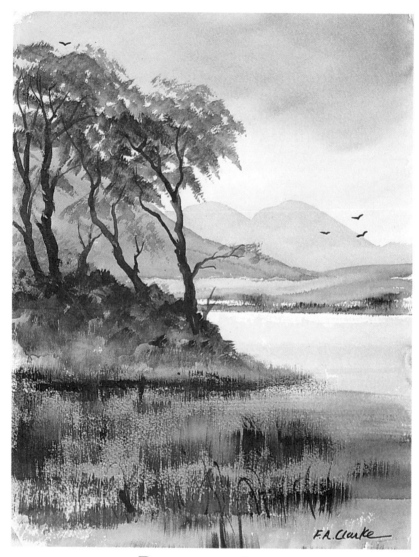

Derryclare Lake

FOR THIS LESSON YOU WILL NEED THE FOLLOWING MATERIALS
1.5" (38MM) WINSOR & NEWTON *Simply Painting* LARGE BRUSH
WINSOR & NEWTON *Simply Painting* SMALL BRUSH
1 SHEET OF 140 LB (300 GSM) WATERCOLOUR PAPER 10" x 14" (25 X 35 CMS)
20" x 16" (50 X 40 CMS) BOARD
CONTAINER OF WATER, PENCIL, CLOTH, RULER, ADHESIVE TAPE.
A HAIRDRYER, IF YOU HAVE ONE.

WATERCOLOUR PAINTS
RAW SIENNA • ULTRAMARINE BLUE • LIGHT RED
LEMON YELLOW HUE • BURNT UMBER

9: Derryclare Lake

The next picture we are going to paint is a lake scene from County Galway called Derryclare Lake. Because the painting is in portrait, which means upright, we are able to concentrate on the trees which are an important part of this picture.

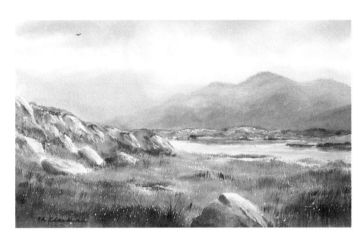

Trees are very scarce in the west of Ireland because sheep eat the small trees. However Derryclare lake has islands which the sheep can't get onto and it's one of these islands we are going to paint.

Step 1: Have - Horizon

This picture is being painted in portrait so the first thing to do is to attach your paper to the board on three sides with a short side at the bottom.

Then draw the horizon line between six and seven inches up from the bottom of the page - just below half way.

Step 2: Some - Sky

On this occasion we want to paint a plain sky, but even so, remember you only have two minutes to paint it. So put out some Ultramarine Blue, Raw Sienna and Light Red on the palette.

With the large brush take some water and wet the paper down to within one inch of the horizon line. Then with Ultramarine Blue only, start at the top of the paper and paint the sky.

Now while the paint is still wet, add a little Light Red to the Ultramarine Blue mixture on your palette and, starting at the top, paint some onto the sky.

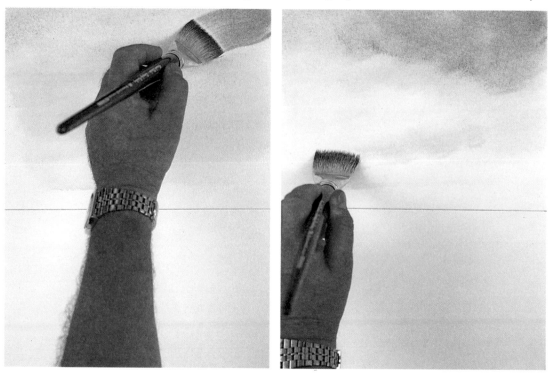

Now let the sky dry, this should only take two minutes.

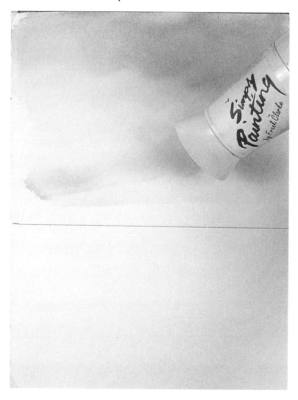

Tip: Only put the paints out as you need them, you don't need the whole palette cluttered up with paints you are not using.

Step 3: More - Middleground

This mountain range is called the Maamturk Mountains. Let's paint the distant mountains first, these are the lightest mountains in the picture.

You can take your time painting the mountains, the two minute rule only applies to the sky.

Use the large brush with 80% Raw Sienna and 20% Ultramarine Blue and with this light mixture, paint the mountains. Now dry the picture well.

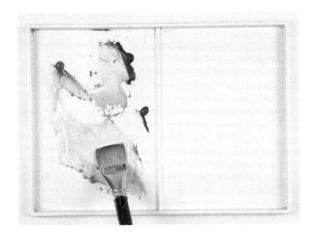

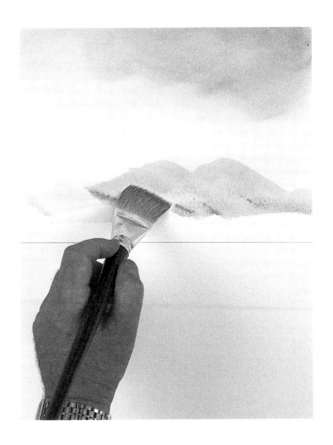
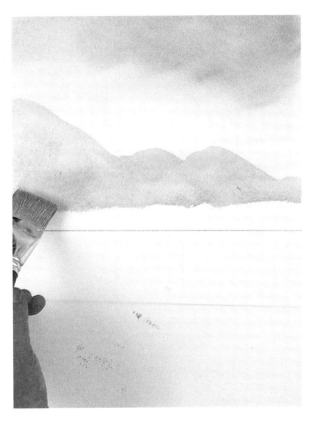

67

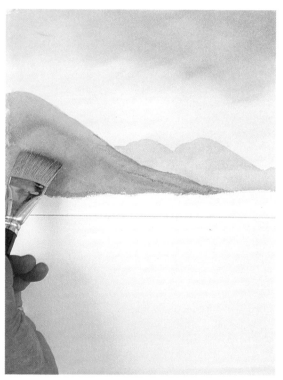

The large mountain is nearer and darker. Do this by painting the large mountain with Ultramarine Blue and a little Light Red, the same mixture you used for the top of the sky.

You will notice that this has the effect of showing the distant mountains in sunlight.

Now we need to paint the middleground between the lake and the mountains, and for this we need to add some Lemon Yellow Hue to our palette.

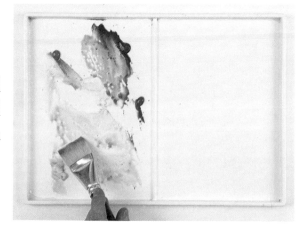

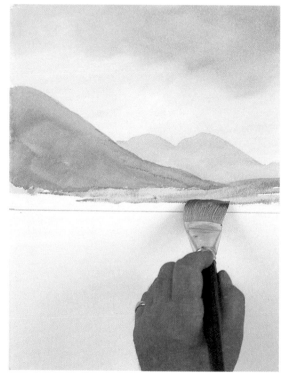

Make a faint green colour with some Lemon Yellow Hue, Raw Sienna and a little Ultramarine Blue and paint the middleground. This mixture is made mostly of Lemon Yellow Hue and remember to keep above the horizon line.

Tip: In watercolour painting mix your colours on the palette, not on the paper.

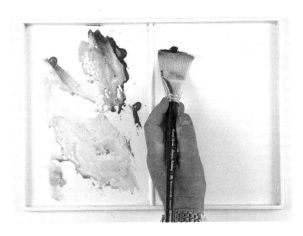

Next squeeze some Burnt Umber onto the palette and, using Burnt Umber only, paint the river bank on the far side of the lake with the large brush using narrow horizontal strokes.

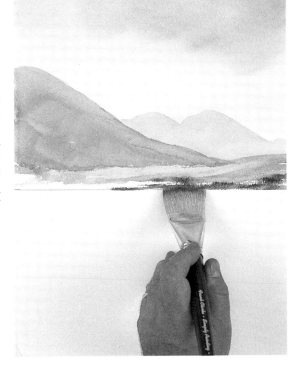

Don't forget to leave the odd gap in the river bank. There is no need to paint all across the horizon line because we going to cover the area on the left with the stand of trees. There now, I have just saved you some paint.

Step 4: Fun - Foreground

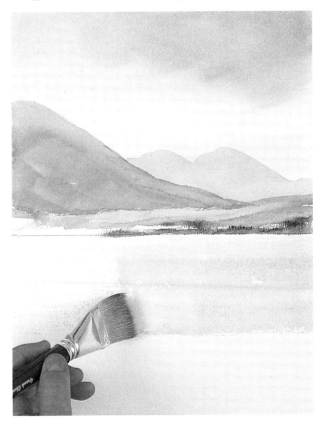

Now let's paint the lake. For this we need a weak mixture of Ultramarine Blue.

Paint the water underneath the horizon line, using the large brush with broad horizontal strokes.

Proceed to within 1" of the bottom of the picture but don't paint the area on the left below the horizon line. Look at the finished picture.

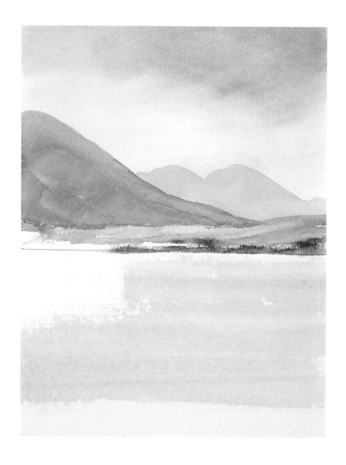

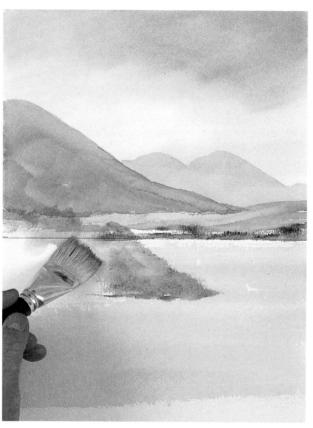

We can now paint the island in the middleground where the trees are growing.

Mix mostly Lemon Yellow Hue, Raw Sienna and a tiny bit of Ultramarine Blue, which gives us a green colour and paint the island.

Paint it with light colours first because in watercolours, we paint from light to dark, and not the other way around.

The bottom of the island should be parallel to the horizon line.

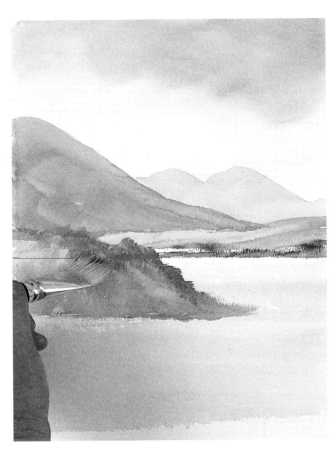

Having done that, add some darker colour to the island with a mixture of Ultramarine Blue and Lemon Yellow Hue and a tiny bit of Raw Sienna.

At this stage dry the picture because if you don't the paint will soak into the wet paint underneath.

Look at the finished picture. Then with Burnt Umber, paint the bottom of the island along the water's edge and the top of the island, leaving a light area in the centre.

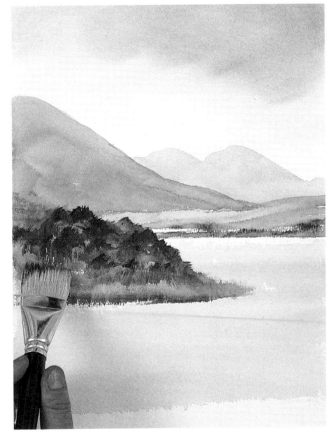

Now on the top of the island, dab in some lighter colour, which is made up of Lemon Yellow Hue and very little Ultramarine Blue.

Next paint the skeletons of the trees. With the small brush and Burnt Umber, start with the one on the right of the bank. Trees grow in different directions, they don't have to be absolutely perfect, so make sure that they don't look like telegraph poles.

Starting from the ground up, draw the small brush upwards. As you paint, lift the brush gently off the paper. This will cause the brush to make thinner branches. Keep doing this until you have completed all the tree skeletons. Don't forget to refer to the finished picture.

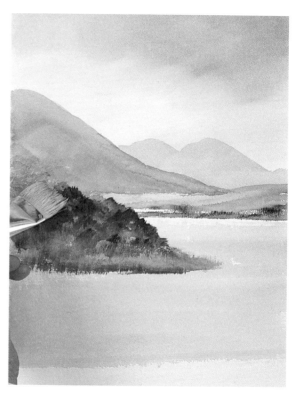

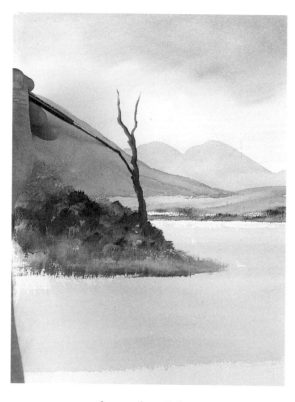
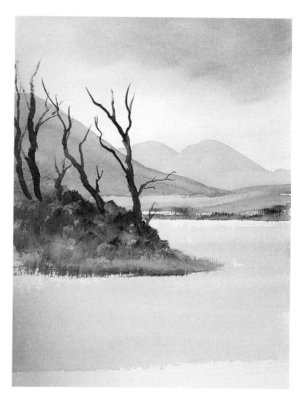

You may wonder why I keep saying, 'look at the finished picture' The fact is, we get so excited with our masterpiece, we forget to look at what we are painting.

Let's paint the leaves of the trees next. This is done with a mixture of Lemon Yellow Hue, Raw Sienna and very little Ultramarine Blue.
Start by painting light colours on the trees first and working to darker colours. Use the corner of the large brush.

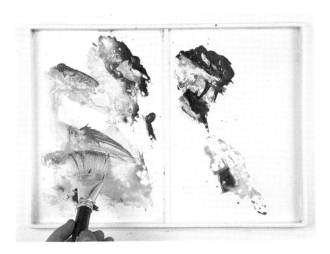

Tip: Make sure the large brush is quite dry when painting the leaves.

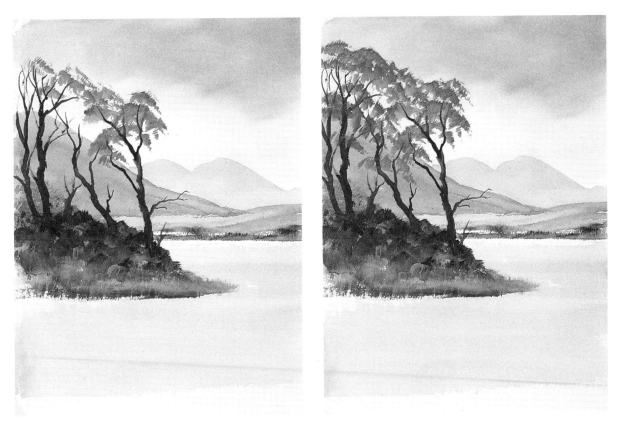

Tip: Each time you pick up paint, make the colour slightly different so that the trees have many different shades.

To make the colours darker add in more Ultramarine Blue.

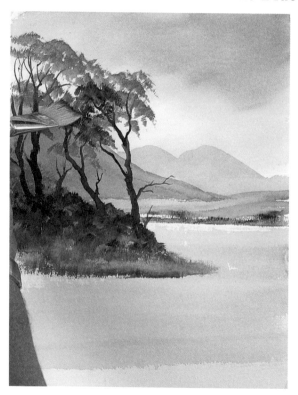

Now when that dries, dab on some neat Lemon Yellow Hue here and there on the outside of the trees to create a light glowing colour. This is done with the corner of the large brush and it needs to be almost dry.

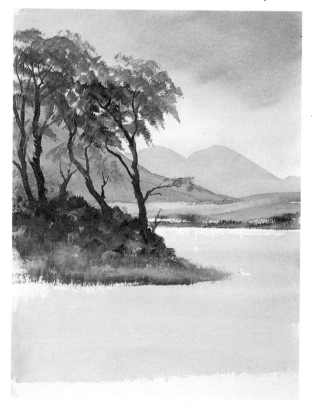

The next thing to do is darken the water on the near side of the island. So take some Ultramarine Blue and paint just below the island exactly as you did for the water below the horizon line. Now once again, let it dry. Use your hairdryer, if you have one otherwise let it dry naturally.

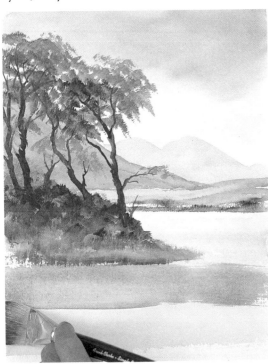
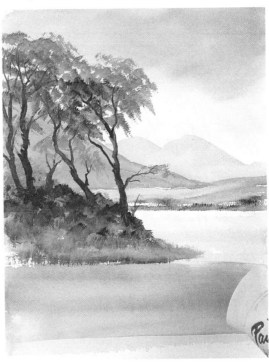

Create some reeds or rushes around the bottom of the island and in the lake using Burnt Umber with downward strokes of the large brush.

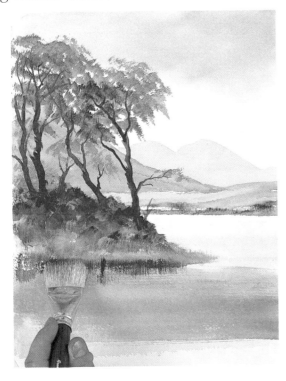
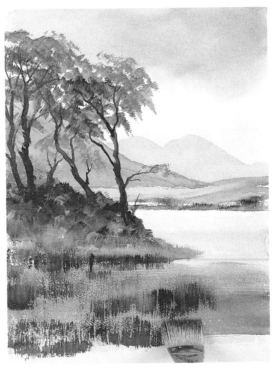

Now paint the river bank nearest us in the foreground. For that we need Lemon Yellow Hue and a tiny bit of Ultramarine Blue to create a light green colour.

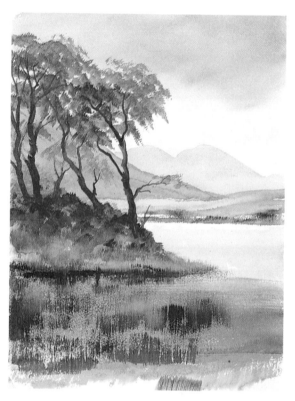

Finish it off by painting some more reeds with the large brush and a little Burnt Umber.

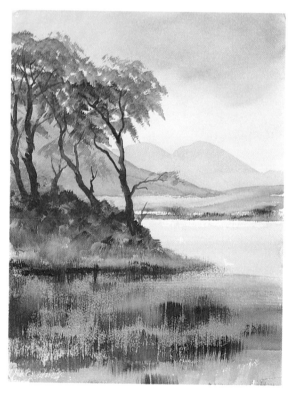

Create a few tall rushes at the bottom of the picture with upwards strokes of the small brush.

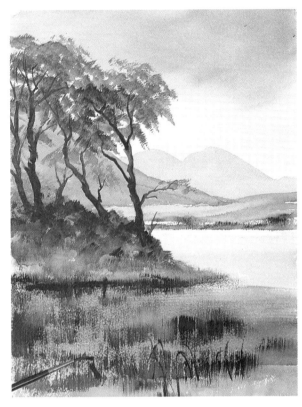

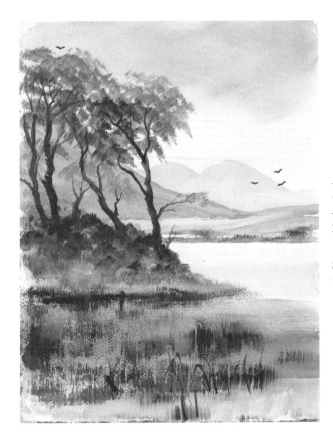

Finally we have reached the stage of painting our bird. If you like, paint one bird in the left hand top corner and some more flying down towards the lake.

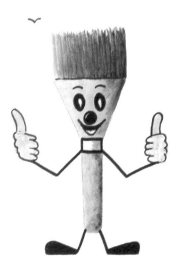

And that completes the picture.

All that's left to do now is to sign it.

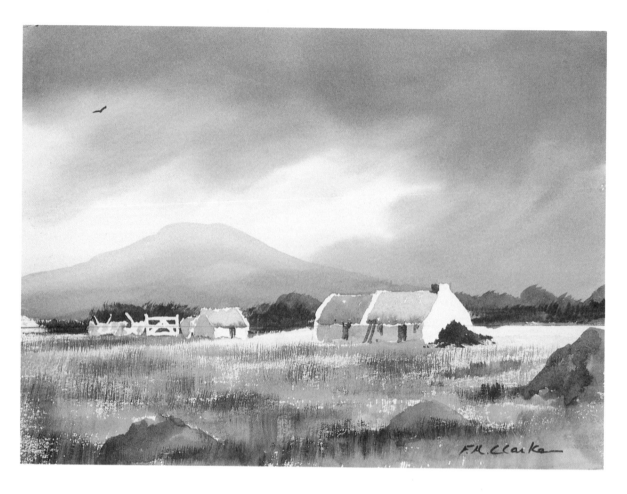

COTTAGES NEAR ROUNDSTONE MOUNTAIN

FOR THIS LESSON YOU WILL NEED THE FOLLOWING MATERIALS
1.5" (38MM) WINSOR & NEWTON *Simply Painting* LARGE BRUSH
WINSOR & NEWTON *Simply Painting* SMALL BRUSH
1 SHEET OF 140 LB (300 GSM) WATERCOLOUR PAPER 10" x 14" (25 X 35 CMS)
MASKING FLUID AND A SMALL CHEAP BRUSH
20" x 16" (50 X 40 CMS) BOARD
CONTAINER OF WATER, PENCIL, CLOTH, RULER, ADHESIVE TAPE.
A HAIRDRYER, IF YOU HAVE ONE.

WATERCOLOUR PAINTS
RAW SIENNA • ULTRAMARINE BLUE • LIGHT RED
LEMON YELLOW HUE • BURNT UMBER

10: Cottages Near Roundstone Mountain

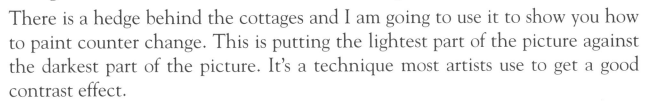

Irish thatched cottages are beautiful and very cosy, I've spent many happy days in them. In this picture we're going to paint some cottages with Roundstone mountain in the background.

There is a hedge behind the cottages and I am going to use it to show you how to paint counter change. This is putting the lightest part of the picture against the darkest part of the picture. It's a technique most artists use to get a good contrast effect.

We will also be using masking fluid so I suggest you read the section on masking fluid (page 12) at the beginning of the book before commencing this picture.

Step 1: Have - Horizon

As we are going to paint this picture in landscape, attach the paper to your board on three sides with a long side at the bottom.

The horizon line is about one-third of the way up the picture, so using your pencil and a ruler draw the horizon line.

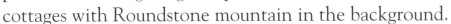

This time we have to do a little more drawing than usual. We have to draw two cottages, a gate and a wall, but it's not difficult when we use the *Simply Painting* method and simplify everything.

So let's begin by drawing the cottage on the right and to start we need to draw two letter V's upside down.

Use your pencil lightly and place them just above the horizon line. Join the two points at the top of the V's together.

Then join the points at the bottom and you have a roof.

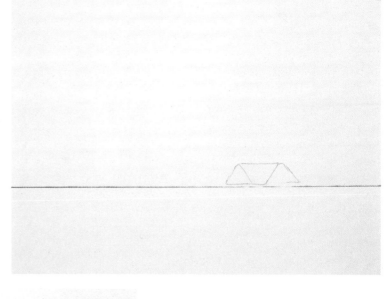

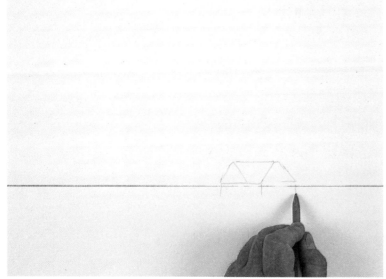

Under the V's draw three legs for the walls of the cottage. These should cross over the horizon line.

Now add another V, slightly smaller than the first ones, at the left of the cottage and join it up with the main cottage.

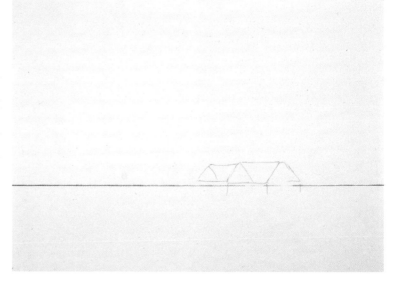

Draw another leg under the V for the wall of the cottage and finish with a chimney on the right hand side of the roof.

That completes the large cottage.

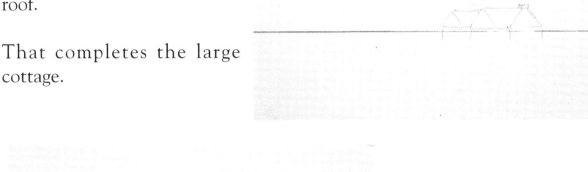

Now, at the left of the cottage draw a smaller cottage. Do it exactly the same way as you did the main house.

Beside the cottage, draw the gate and then the wall. You don't have to draw these exactly as I have them, they are only a guide. If you make a mistake, don't worry just use your eraser to remove it and start again.

Now having completed all the drawing, let's paint them with masking fluid.

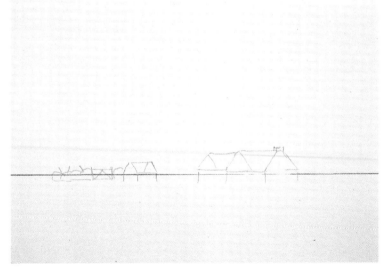

You will notice the masking fluid is a yellow colour. I prefer it because you can see it on the paper.

Get a small cheap brush and dip it in water, don't use one of your good brushes, as the masking fluid can damage it.

Then, holding the masking fluid firmly, being careful it doesn't spill, paint the cottage and the little stores beside it with masking fluid.

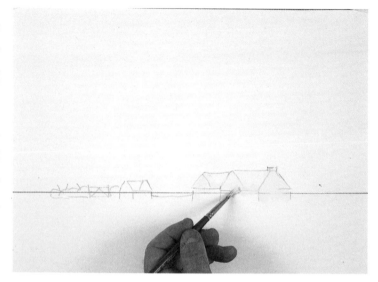

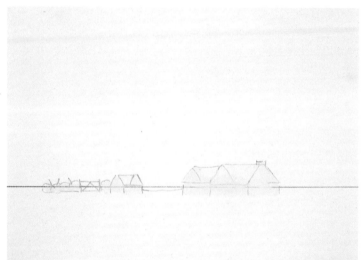

Now paint the gate, but only the bars of the gate, and the walls on the left and right of it.

Then very carefully put the top back on your masking fluid and wash your brush in the water.

Now let the masking fluid you have just painted dry thoroughly because if you don't, your brushes will stick to it when you are painting the sky.

It will take about ten minutes for the masking fluid to dry, so why not treat yourself to a cup of coffee.

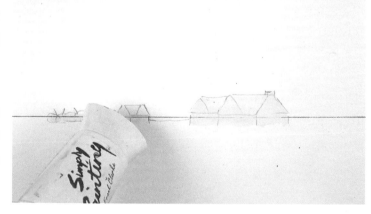

82

Step2: Some - Sky

Let's concentrate on the sky now. Squeeze out some Raw Sienna, Ultramarine Blue and Light Red onto the side of your palette. With the large brush, take some of the Raw Sienna into the centre of your palette. Starting from the top of the paper, paint the background right down to the horizon line. Don't use too much paint in the mixture, we just want a light wash on the paper.

While the sky is still wet, take some Ultramarine Blue to the centre of the palette and paint a coat of blue over the sky. Keep the colour dark at the bottom, because the darker it is the better the counter change will work.

Counter change sounds complicated, but it's not, it just means putting dark against light. All professions use phrases which people outside the profession don't understand, but then that's the whole idea.

This time leave some of the sky unpainted so that the Raw Sienna shows through. Refer to the finished painting.

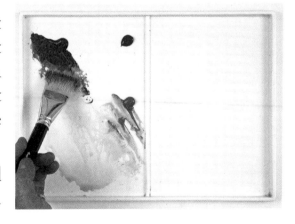

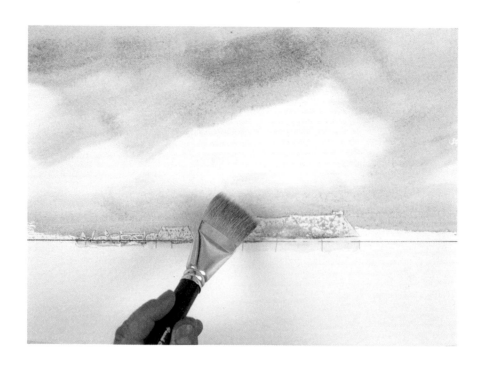

Now add a little Light Red to the Ultramarine Blue on the palette and paint the sky while it is still wet.

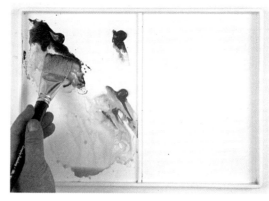

Let the picture dry, use your hairdryer or wait until it is completely dry before starting to paint again.

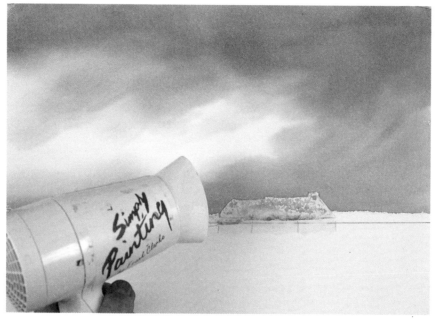

Step 3: More - Middleground

Next, let's paint the mountain in the background. In this case it is only half of the letter M. Using the large brush with a mixture of Ultramarine Blue and Light Red, make the same colour as you did for the darkest part of the sky.

Start just above the horizon line ignoring the cottage and paint the mountain. What I mean by this is you can paint over the cottages as the masking fluid will protect them. Next dry it using a hairdryer or wait until it is dry before continuing.

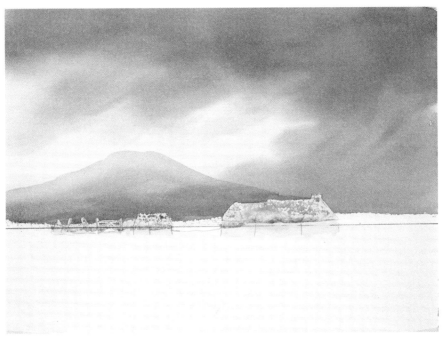

Now we are ready to create the counter change in the picture. First put some Lemon Yellow Hue and Burnt Umber on the palette.

Using Lemon Yellow Hue and Raw Sienna with a little Ultramarine Blue, paint the bushes and trees along the horizon line. Don't worry about painting over the cottages as they are well protected by the masking fluid.

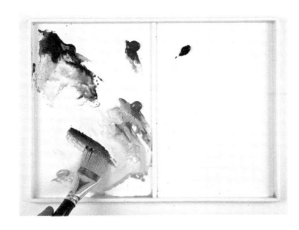

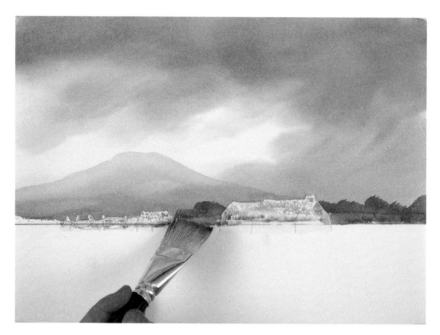

Add a little extra Ultramarine Blue to the mixture to darken it slightly and that completes our counter change.

Now dry the picture well.

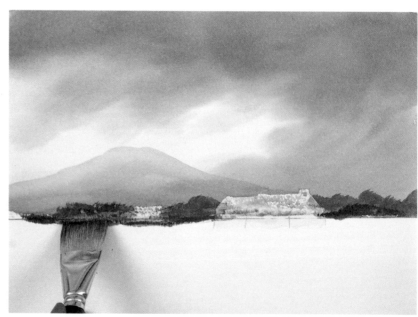

Step 4: Fun - Foreground

Next let's paint the grass below the horizon line. Make a weak mixture of Raw Sienna, that is, using more water on the palette.

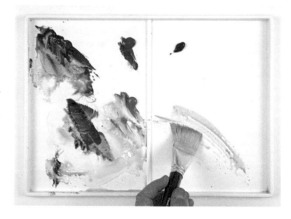

Paint the foreground to about 2" from the bottom of the paper. Use the large brush with broad horizontal strokes.

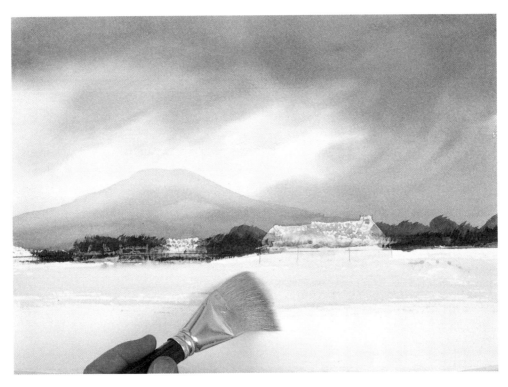

Using a mixture of Lemon Yellow Hue, Raw Sienna and Ultramarine Blue, create some grass in the foreground with downward strokes of the large brush. Use mostly Lemon Yellow Hue.

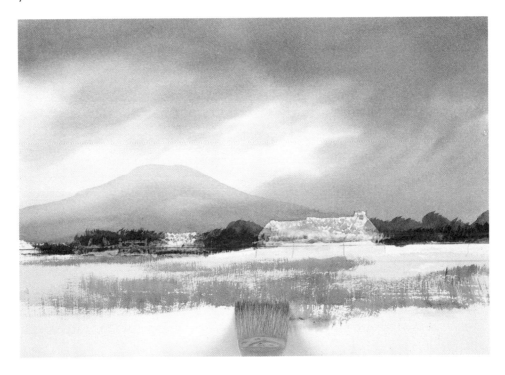

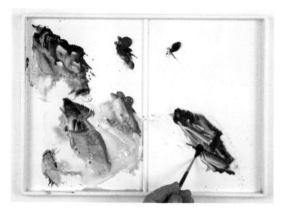

Next paint the rocks using the small brush with Ultramarine Blue, a little bit of Light Red and some Raw Sienna.

Mix them thoroughly together on the palette to make a grey shade. To lighten it add more Raw Sienna and to darken it add more Ultramarine Blue.

Tip: Try out the mixture on a spare sheet of paper.

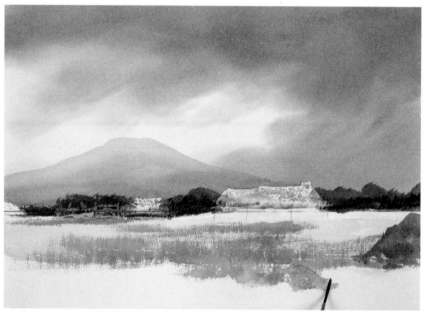

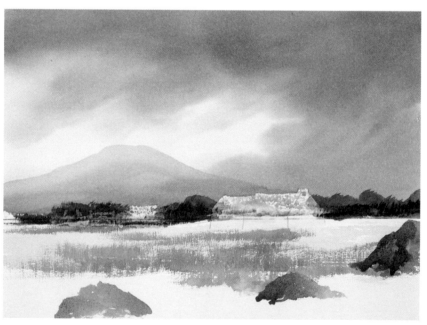

Add in some shadows here and there on the rocks using a darker mixture.

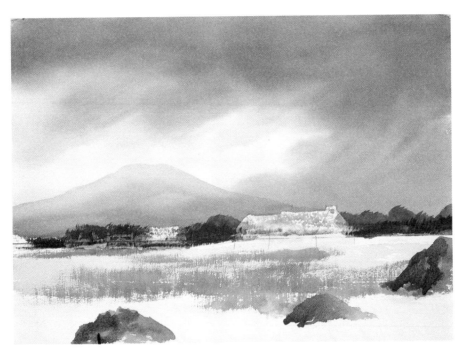

Then dry the rocks with your hairdryer or wait until they are completely dry before painting the rest of the foreground.

Now with a mixture of Lemon Yellow Hue, Raw Sienna, and Ultramarine Blue using downward strokes of the large brush, paint the foreground around and below the rocks. Make it a darker mixture than the grass by using more Ultramarine Blue.

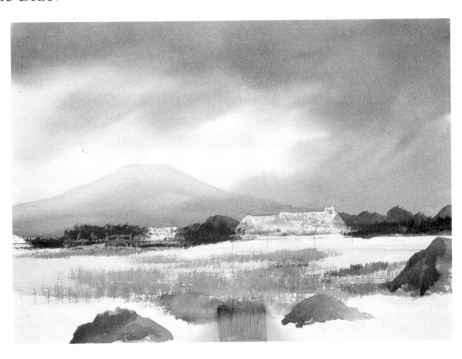

Then with only Burnt Umber on the brush, use downward strokes to create the grassy effect at the bottom of the picture. You can paint over the bottom of the rocks to anchor them into the ground. That completes the foreground.

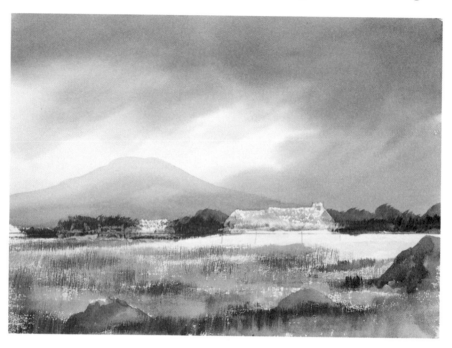

Now it's time to go back to the cottages and the gate. So, take a rubber or an eraser and rub off the masking fluid, being careful to rub from the edges of the masking fluid towards the centre of the area which is protected. The reason we rub towards the centre is that if the paper tears, it won't damage the background behind the cottage.

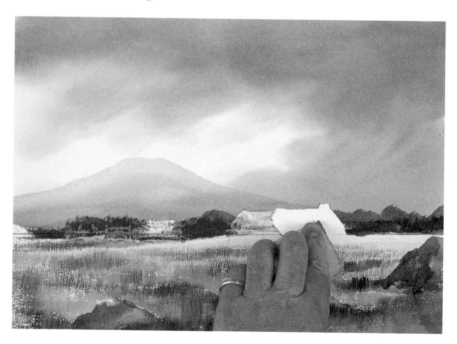

WOW we have a perfect outline of the cottages, the wall and the gate and it's in counter change.

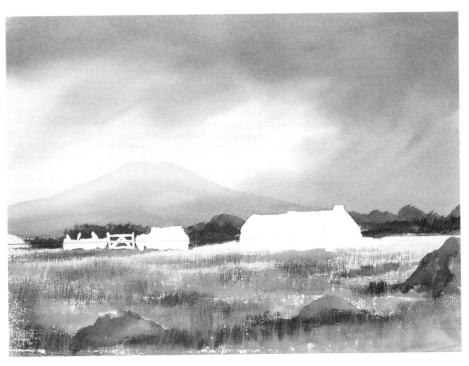

Having removed all the masking fluid, let's paint the roofs of the cottages. Starting with the big cottage on the right hand side and using some Raw Sienna with a tiny bit of Burnt Umber and the small brush, paint the roof of the cottage.

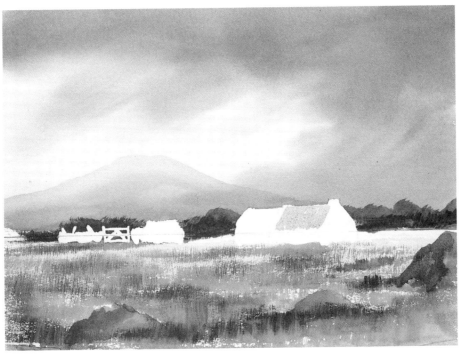

The roof of the lean-to connected to the main cottage is older, so when painting it add some extra Burnt Umber to make it darker. Now at the bottom of both roofs, just dab on some Burnt Umber only and this will give the impression of depth to the roofs.

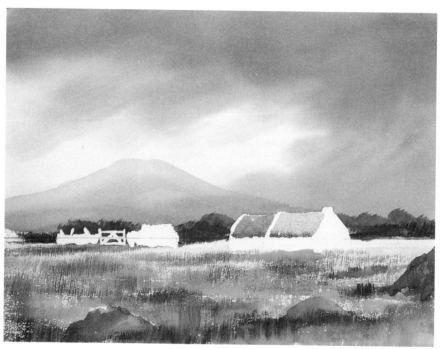

Now paint the roof of the cottage on the left hand side, the one beside the gate, doing the same thing except using lighter paint, because after all it is facing directly into the sun.

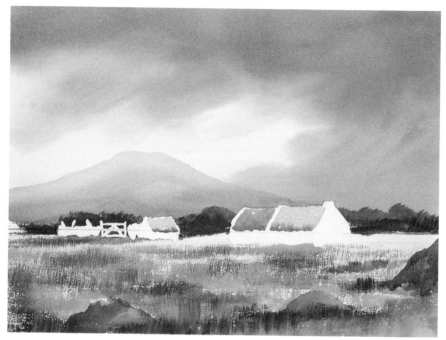

I hope you keep referring to the finished picture.

Now, before painting the walls of the cottages which are in shadow, dry the roofs. First paint the front wall of the large cottage and then the gable end of the small cottage. Use the small brush and a mixture of Light Red and Ultramarine Blue with plenty of water to make the colour weak.

Tip: It's a good idea to test this shadow colour on a piece of scrap paper before you start to paint it.

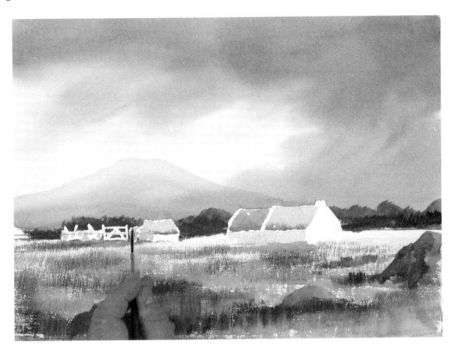

If the shadow is not dark enough don't add more paint, just dry the cottages and paint over them with the same colour. This will double the density of shadow.

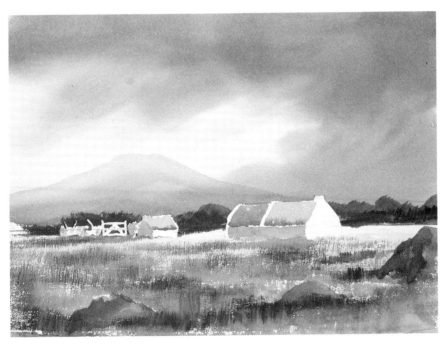

We are now going to create a dark colour for the doors and windows of the cottages. This is done with a mixture of Ultramarine Blue and Burnt Umber.

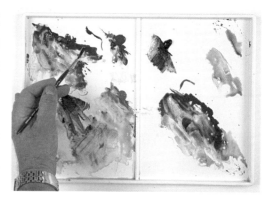

Paint the doors with a couple of narrow downward strokes with the small brush and paint the windows with shorter strokes.

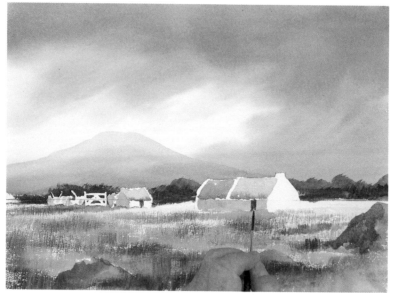

Now shade the left hand side of the chimney using the small brush and Burnt Umber only. Paint two lengths of wood lying up against the wall of the cottage with the same mixture.

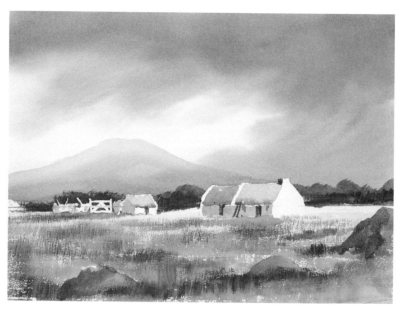

Lastly, there is a pile of turf which we call a rick, at the gable end of the large cottage.

To paint this rick of turf use short strokes with the small brush and Burnt Umber.

Finally, there are just two things left to do, one is to paint the bird, and the last thing is to sign it.

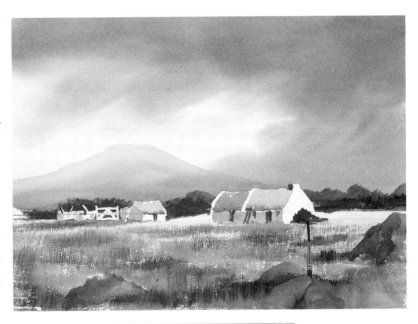

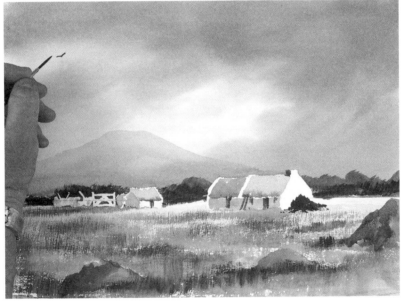

Well done, another masterpiece!

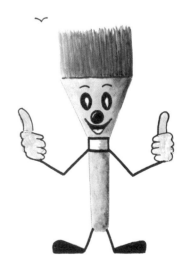

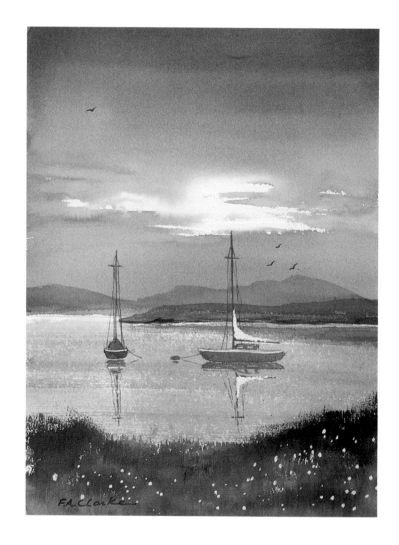

BOATS IN THE EVENING AT CLIFDEN BAY

FOR THIS LESSON YOU WILL NEED THE FOLLOWING MATERIALS
1.5" (38MM) WINSOR & NEWTON *Simply Painting* LARGE BRUSH
WINSOR & NEWTON *Simply Painting* SMALL BRUSH
1 SHEET OF 140 LB (300 GSM) WATERCOLOUR PAPER 10" x 14" (25 X 35 CMS)
20" x 16" (50 X 40 CM) BOARD

CONTAINER OF WATER, PENCIL, CLOTH, RULER, ADHESIVE TAPE.
A HAIRDRYER, IF YOU HAVE ONE.

WATERCOLOUR PAINTS

RAW SIENNA • ULTRAMARINE BLUE • LIGHT RED • LEMON YELLOW HUE
BURNT UMBER • ALIZARIN CRIMSON • DESIGNER'S WHITE GOUACHE

11: Boats in the Evening at Clifden Bay

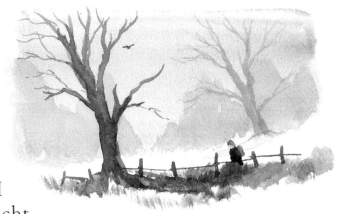

Let's look at the finished picture we are going to paint. It is a sunset scene just outside the town of Clifden in the west of Ireland. I went for a walk to the Clifden Yacht Club and by the time I got there, the sun was setting and the sky was a purpley pink. There were two boats anchored in the bay and I thought the scene would make a lovely subject.

Before we start let me tell you a little about artistic license. What's that? Well if there is something in a scene that you don't like, you can change it or leave it out. In this scene one boat was blue and the other was red. I decided to make both boats the same colour because in a sunset scene like this, it would look silly to have a bright blue boat and a bright red boat. Having said that, off we go.

Step 1: Have - Horizon

Once again we are painting in portrait, so using some adhesive tape, attach your paper to the board on three sides with a short side at the bottom.

Then with your pencil and ruler, draw the horizon line about six inches (152mm) up from the bottom of the page.

Make sure the horizon line is straight, because if it's not the sea will look very strange. There are no hills in the ocean.

Step 2: Some - Sky

Look at the finished picture, there is a little light in the centre where the sun is going down behind the clouds. As I have said before, in watercolours we paint from light to dark, that is, we paint light colours first and then dark colours.

Let's start by painting the yellow in the centre which is surrounding the sun.

Squeeze some Lemon Yellow Hue, Alizarin Crimson and Ultramarine Blue onto the side of your palette.

For this picture you <u>don't</u> need to wet the paper before you start to paint the sky.

With the large brush add some water to the Lemon Yellow Hue on the palette and paint a light mixture of yellow in the centre of the sky only.

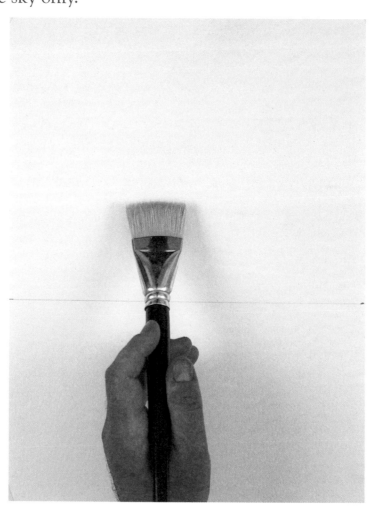

98

Now add some Alizarin Crimson to the yellow mixture on your palette and starting from the top of the paper, which is dry, paint the rest of the sky down to the horizon line.

Take care to paint around the yellow in the centre. This gives the effect of sunlight radiating through the clouds.

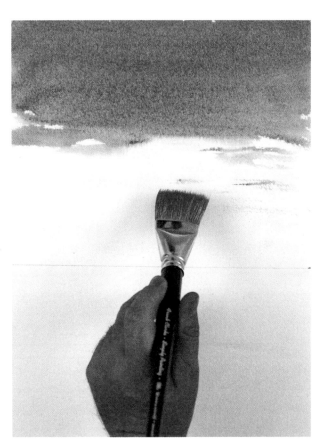

Remember the two minute rule applies.

If you don't know what the two minute rule is you didn't read the start of the book, so back you go to page 21 The Two Minute Sky.

Next add some Ultramarine Blue to the Lemon Yellow Hue and Alizarin Crimson mixture on your palette and paint some of this darker colour at the top of the sky.

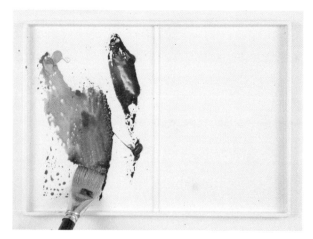

You can also add a tiny amount to the bottom of the sky. When you are finished, dry the picture and that completes the sky.

Step 3: More - Middleground

In this picture the sky is red and so too are the mountains because they reflect the colours of the sky. It would be silly to have green mountains with a red sky. It is really only a matter of observation isn't it?

So, let's paint the distant mountains. Once again use the large brush and a mixture of Lemon Yellow Hue with a little Alizarin Crimson and Ultramarine Blue. These are of course, the same colours we used to paint the sky.

100

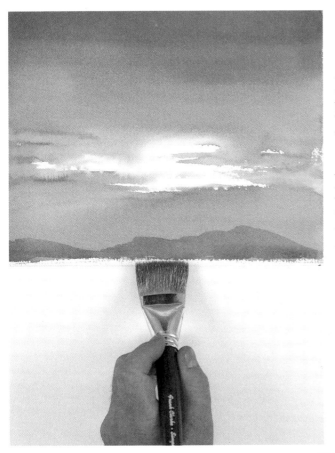

Paint a flat letter M just above the horizon line using the large brush with narrow horizontal strokes.

Now dry the picture. Use your hairdryer if you have one, otherwise wait until it has dried completely before you continue.

Now with the same colours, we are going to create the headland near us, except this time use a little more Ultramarine Blue in the mixture.

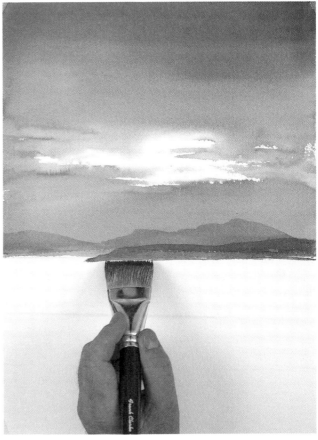

It is important that the bottom of the headland, which is underneath the horizon line, is parallel to the horizon line.

Check it with your ruler and if it is not straight, straighten it by filling in with more paint.

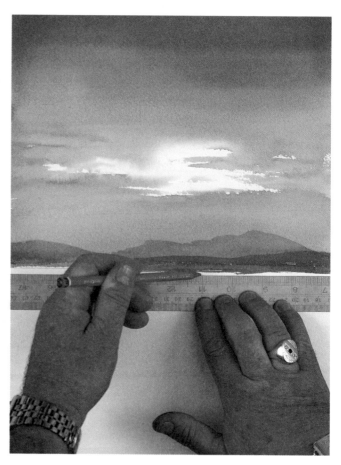

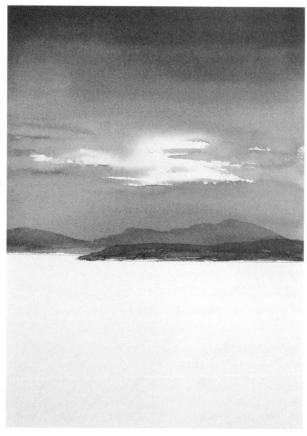

Now, once more let it dry or dry it with the hairdryer.

Step 4: Fun - Foreground

Next we are going to paint the sea with a light mixture of Alizarin Crimson, Ultramarine Blue and a tiny bit of Lemon Yellow Hue.
Use equal amounts of Alizarin Crimson and Ultramarine Blue.

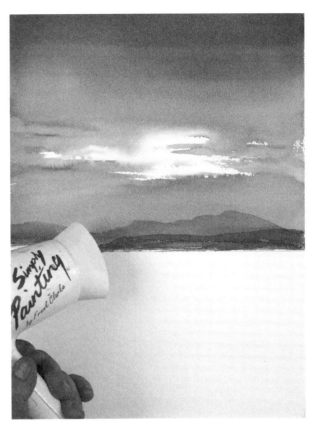

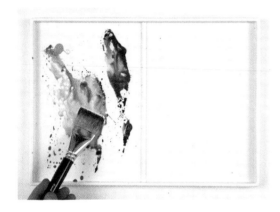

Use broad horizontal strokes with the large brush and don't stop when you're painting the water.

Continue your stroke right across the paper otherwise you'll get brush marks in your picture.

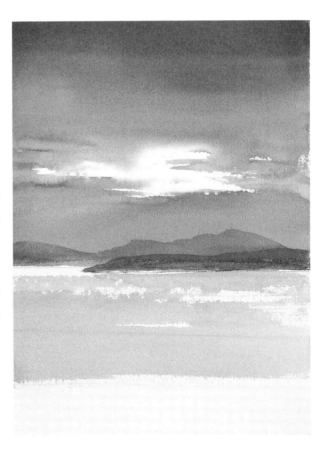

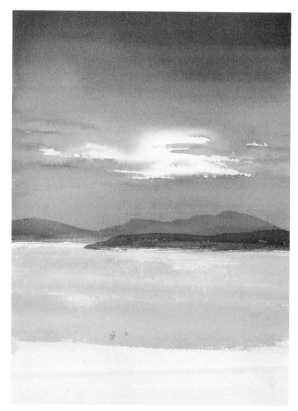

Now let the sea dry or dry it with your hairdryer.

In the sea, paint a shadow below the headland, using the small brush with a weak mixture of Ultramarine Blue and Alizarin Crimson.

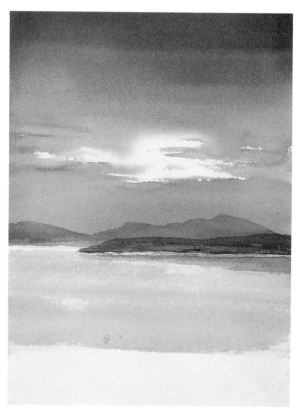

Now squeeze some Burnt Umber onto the side of your palette. At the bottom of the headland where it meets the sea, paint some Burnt Umber with the small brush. This gives the impression of a rocky shore on the headland.

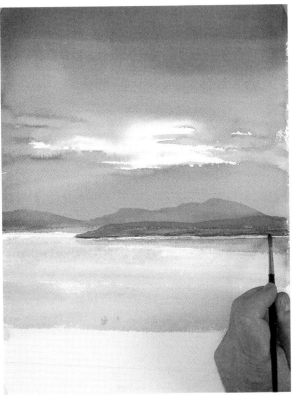

I would prefer the sea to be a little darker, to reflect more of the colour in the sky.

To darken it I am going to paint over it again with the same colour I used to paint the sea in the first place and this will automatically double the density of the paint. But first the painting must be completely dry.

So with the large brush, in exactly the same way you painted the sea in the first place, paint the water again.

This may not be necessary if, unlike me, you get it right first time.

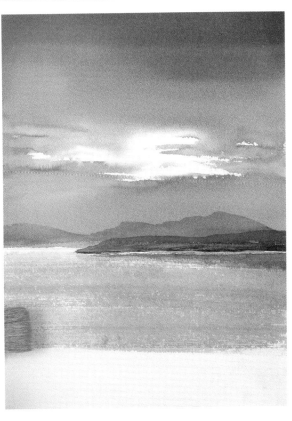

105

Next look at the boats in the finished picture. There are two boats, the nearest one is broadside to us and the other we can see end on. Let's start with the one which is nearest. It is about 1 1/2" (38mm) below the headland and the bottom of it will be parallel to the horizon line.

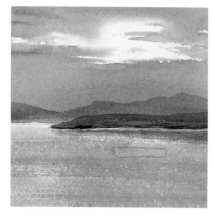

How do you paint boats? Well using your pencil, draw a rectangle. It's a good idea to practice this on a sheet of paper first.

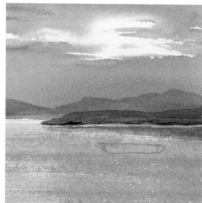

Then add the ends on it.

Finally put the wheel-house on.

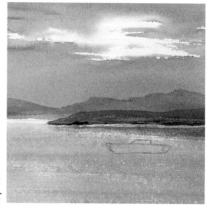

Next we are going to draw the second boat. It looks like the letter U, so draw the letter U to the left of the first boat.

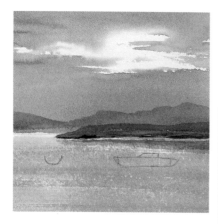

Tip: To give the impression of the boat being further away, it should be nearer the horizon line.

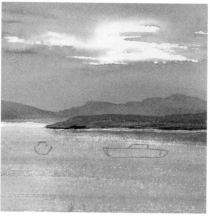

Then add the wheel house, which in this case is only a flat U upside down.

All that is left to do is draw the masts and we can use the ruler and a pencil for these.

The mast of the first boat is just in front of the wheel house and it extends up just underneath the light part of the sky.

The second boat has a shorter mast because it's a smaller boat and is further away than the first one.

Now let's paint the hulls with Raw Sienna and a little bit of Burnt Umber, so put out some Raw Sienna on the side of your palette.

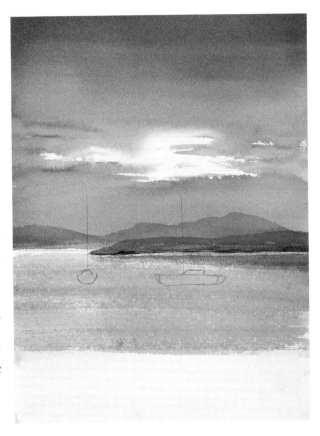

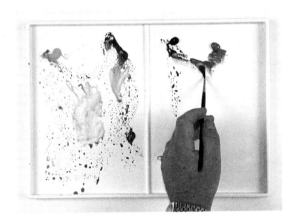

Mix some Raw Sienna and Burnt Umber with the small brush and paint the hull of the large boat.

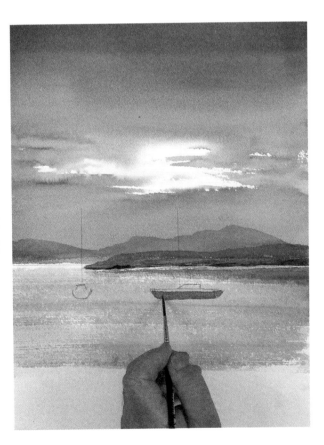

Then paint the hull of small boat and the wheel houses of both boats.

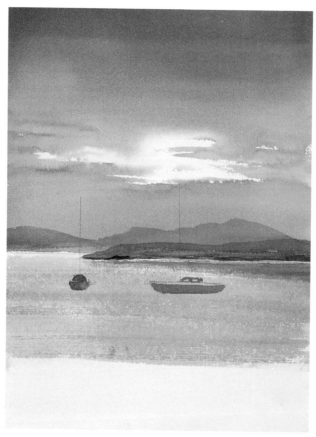

Using the same colour paint the buoy between the boats and a rope leading down into the water from the small boat.

At this stage the painting is looking a little flat but you will be amazed how a few details will change all that.

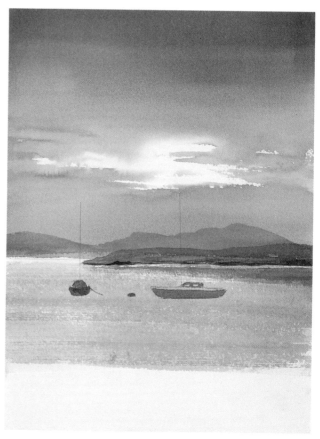

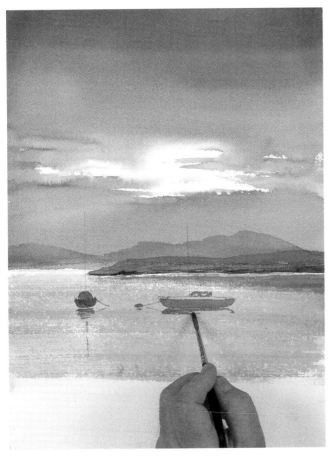

Using the small brush with some Raw Sienna and Burnt Umber, the same colours we used for the hulls of the boats, paint the shadows of the small boat with its mast.

The reflection of the mast is broken by the movement of the water. To represent this, use a broken line when painting the reflection on the water.

Then do the same with the large boat and the buoy.

We drew the masts originally with a ruler and pencil, well on that pencil line I want you to paint some Burnt Umber with your small brush.

Don't be afraid, you can do it. Just hold the small brush as you would a pencil.

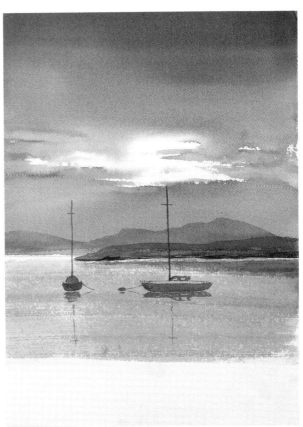

When you have completed that, paint some guide ropes, which are the ropes used to support the mast.

You can if you wish, draw the guide wires on the boats with a ruler, but don't overdo it

Also paint a gib on the large boat extending from the mast towards the back of the boat.

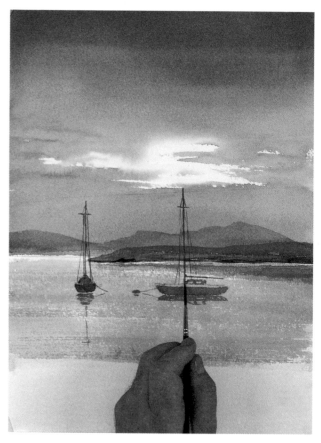

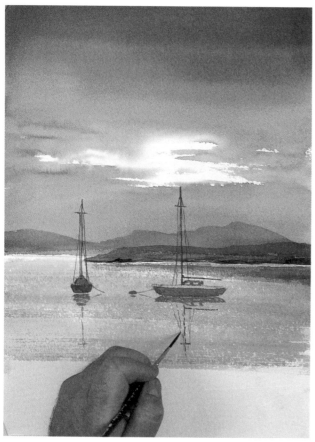

Draw the shadow of the large boat's guide ropes in the water using the small brush and Burnt Umber only.

Remember to paint a broken line.

To create a mottled look in the foreground use Lemon Yellow Hue, Alizarin Crimson and Raw Sienna which gives it a light colour. Then with a mixture of Burnt Umber and Ultramarine Blue create some darker areas and that completes the foreground.

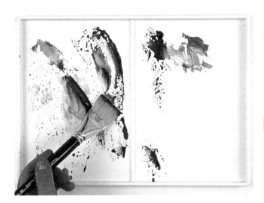 

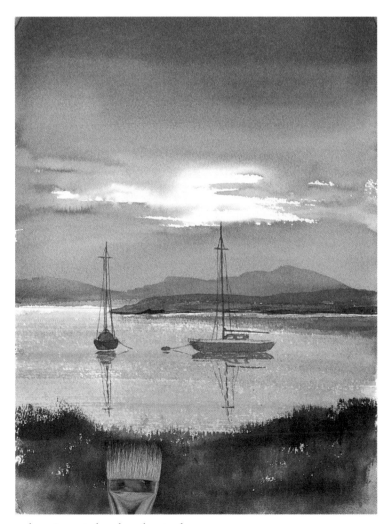

Now, let it dry or dry it with the hairdryer.

To finish the painting let's put sails on the boats and some daisies or bog cotton in the foreground. First put out some White Gouache on the palette and paint the sails on the boats and the top edge of the hull of each boat with the small brush.

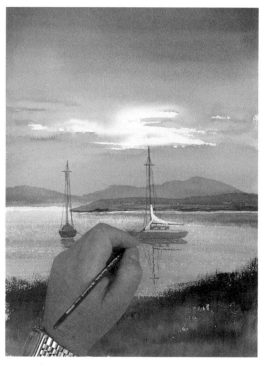

Now, as we have a sail on the boat we must have it reflected in the water. So do that.

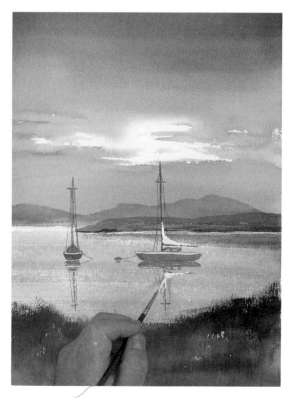

Lastly we need to put some white flowers in the foreground with White Gouache. Just dab it on here and there.

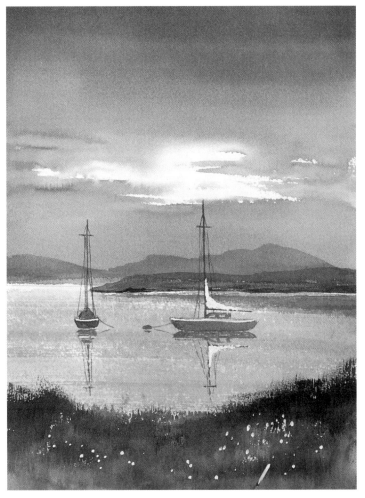

Finally take the small brush and paint the bird with Burnt Umber.

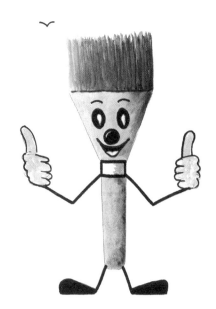

Congratulations.

Now sign your painting.

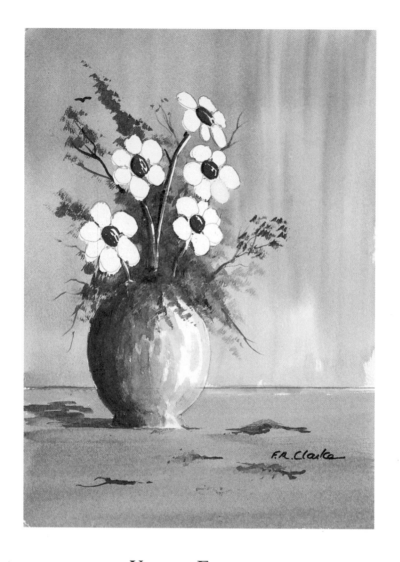

VASE OF FLOWERS

FOR THIS LESSON YOU WILL NEED THE FOLLOWING MATERIALS
1.5" (38MM) WINSOR & NEWTON *Simply Painting* LARGE BRUSH
WINSOR & NEWTON *Simply Painting* SMALL BRUSH
1 SHEET OF 140 LB (300 GSM) WATERCOLOUR PAPER 10" x 14" (25 X 35 CMS)
MASKING FLUID AND A SMALL CHEAP BRUSH
20" X 16" (50 X 40 CMS) BOARD
CONTAINER OF WATER, PENCIL, CLOTH, RULER, ADHESIVE TAPE.
A HAIRDRYER, IF YOU HAVE ONE.

WATERCOLOUR PAINTS
RAW SIENNA • COBALT BLUE HUE • LIGHT RED
LEMON YELLOW HUE • BURNT UMBER • PAYNE'S GRAY
ALIZARIN CRIMSON

114

11: Vase of Flowers

Painting flowers is very easy, and you'll love it. It's also very relaxing because you can set up a scene and paint at home without worrying about the weather or searching for an interesting subject outdoors.

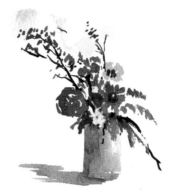

We are going to paint some white flowers which are on a table near a window. I've kept them very simple, but you can paint them any colour you like.

Step 1: Have - Horizon

A portrait shape is always good for flowers, so attach your paper to the board with tape on three sides only, making sure there is a short side at the bottom.

Using your pencil, draw the horizon line which in this case is about 1/3 of the way up from the bottom of the page.

Have a look at the finished picture. You will notice that the only thing which breaks the horizon line is the vase. Also both the vase and flowers are slightly to the left because we don't want to put the main subject of interest directly in the centre of the picture.

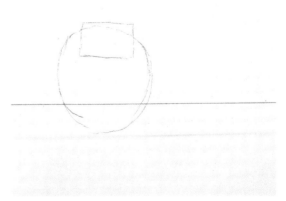

Let's begin by drawing the flowers and the vase. The vase is a circle with a rectangle on top and the flowers consist of an inner circle surrounded by six circles. One of the flowers is flat.

First draw the circle for the vase starting above the horizon line and coming down to break the horizon line. Next draw the rectangle at the top of the vase.

115

Draw a straight line below the vase for it to stand on. Join the straight line to the bottom of the vase and that completes the vase.

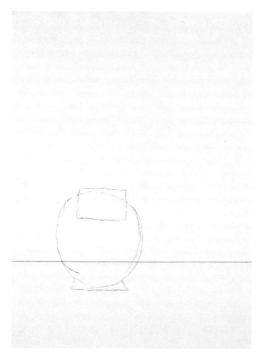

Now there are five flowers all above the horizon line. Place a dot where you want the centre of each flower to be and when you have done this surround each dot with a circle to represent the flower's centre. Remember these are freehand, they do not have to be perfect. The top flower is a flat circle.

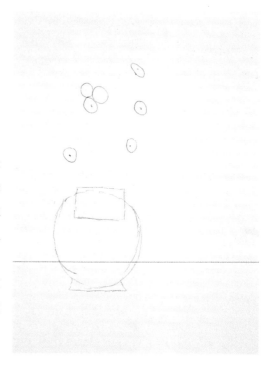

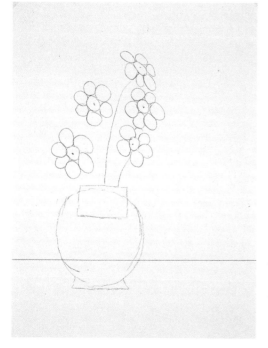

Having done that we now need to put six circles around each of the flower centres.

The circles around the top flower are slightly flattened because the flower is facing upwards.

When we have all five flowers surrounded by circles, draw stems down into the vase.

116

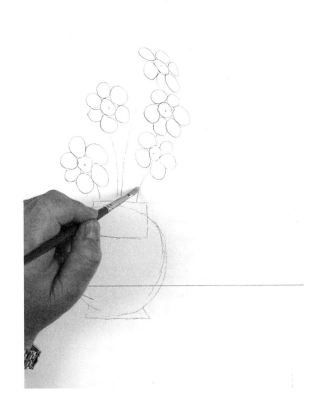

That completes the drawing for this picture. The next thing to do is to protect the flowers, the stems and the vase with masking fluid. So take a cheap brush with the masking fluid and fill in all the circles (see the section on Masking Fluid).

Make sure you also cover the stems and, of course, the vase.

Tip: Start with the circle at the top so you don't stick your elbow or arm into the masking fluid.

After every 20 seconds or so to dip your brush into the water and swish it around to prevent it becoming stiff and covered with masking fluid.

Now clean your brush and let the picture dry. This will take ten minutes or so, have a break, you've done well.

Step 2: Some - Sky

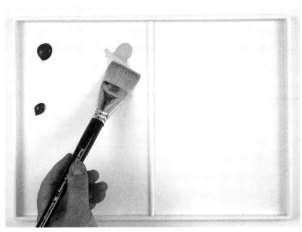

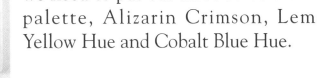

We can now paint the background ignoring the flowers and vase. For this we need to put out three colours on the palette, Alizarin Crimson, Lemon Yellow Hue and Cobalt Blue Hue.

117

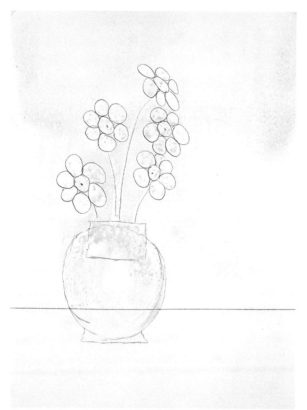

Take the large brush dip it into the water and starting with Lemon Yellow Hue, paint the background.

Paint the whole picture down to the horizon line, ignoring the flowers, you can paint over them, the masking fluid will protect them.

When you have completed that, add some Alizarin Crimson to the mix on your palette and paint the background again.

Use the large brush with broad downward strokes starting on the right hand side and paint down as far as the horizon line.

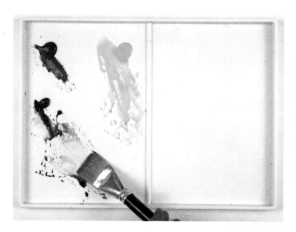

Having completed that, add some Cobalt Blue Hue to the mix and, starting this time from the left hand side of the picture, create a dark side on the left of the picture.

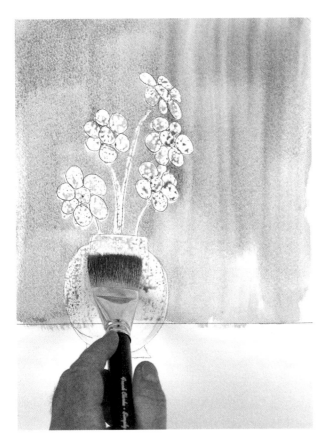

Again use broad downward strokes but only paint to the centre of the picture.

This will give you a shaded finish which runs from Lemon Yellow Hue on the right across to a purple colour on the left.

Tip: Don't fiddle with the background, the two minute rule applies, the same as the sky.

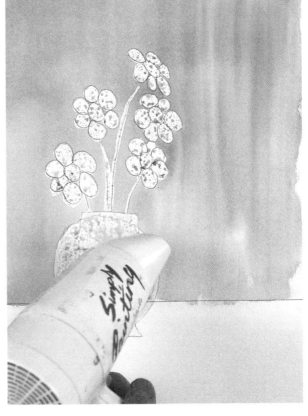

Now that completes the background, put your brush into the water and dry the picture.

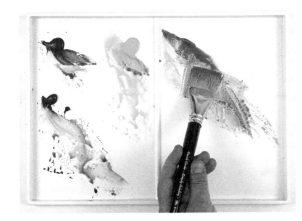

Squeeze some Raw Sienna onto the side of your palette. Now with the large brush make a mixture of 75% Raw Sienna and 25% Alizarin Crimson.

With this mixture paint the bottom of the picture below the vase and dry it again. This is done with broad horizontal brush strokes.

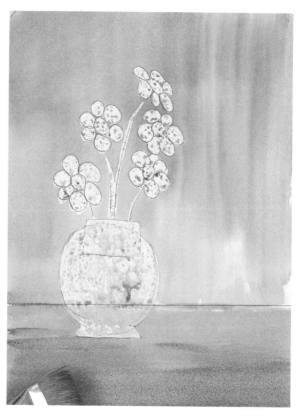

Step 3: More - Middleground

Now before we remove the masking fluid let's paint the background foliage.

Starting with light colours mix some Lemon Yellow Hue and Cobalt Blue Hue to make a light green. Make sure the brush is not too wet, then dab it on with the corner of the large brush.

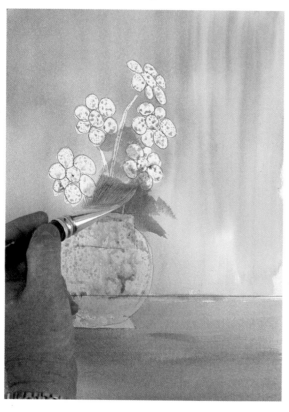

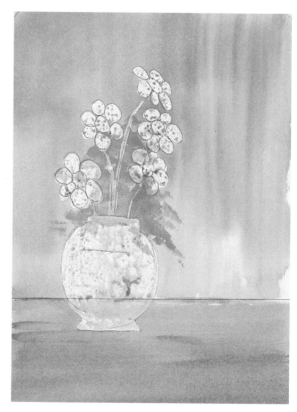

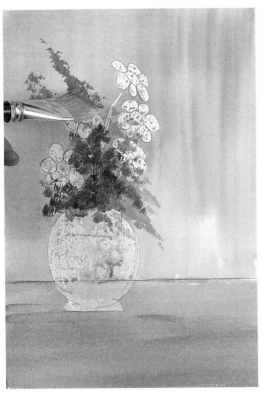

Put out some Payne's Gray on the palette. Mix some Lemon Yellow Hue with a little Alizarin Crimson and very little Payne's Gray and dab the foliage on. Be careful with Payne's Gray because it is a very strong colour.

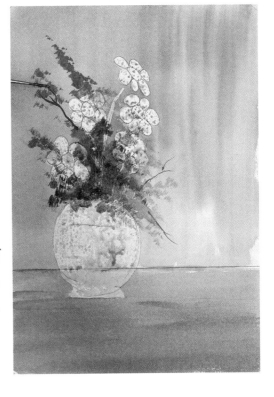

Mix a little of the green, which is made up of the Lemon Yellow Hue and Cobalt Blue Hue with the Payne's Gray and draw some stems. This begins to bring the picture to life.

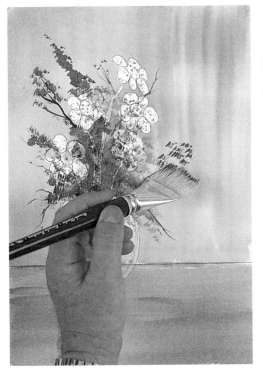

Once again with the corner of the large brush and Alizarin Crimson dab on some flowers, lightly on the right hand side of the flowers.

Now dry the picture very well because anything that isn't dry when we rub off the masking fluid will mark the white paper underneath. If you haven't got a hairdryer why not have a cup of coffee or take a half hour break?

121

When it is perfectly dry, rub off the masking fluid with your finger or an eraser. Be careful, start from the outside and rub towards the centre of the protected area. First rub the masking fluid off the flowers and the stems.

You should now have clean flowers with all the stems visible. In some cases you may find that the paint has managed to sneak through the masking fluid into the background, this doesn't matter just leave it there and it will look quite natural.

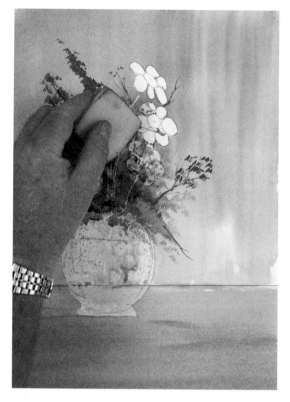

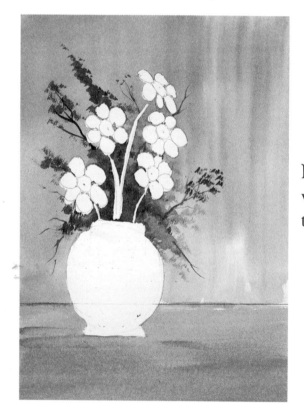

Now rub off the masking fluid from the vase starting from the outside and working towards the centre.

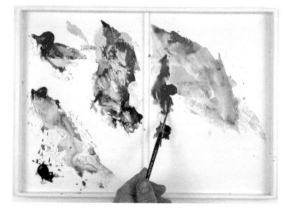

Next with the small brush starting from the top, let's paint the centre of the flowers using Light Red and some Burnt Umber.

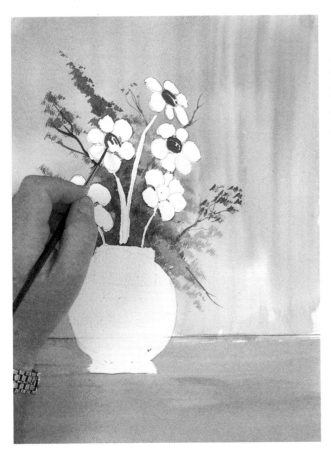

Leave a little paper unpainted on the right of the centre of each flower which will show which direction the light is coming from.

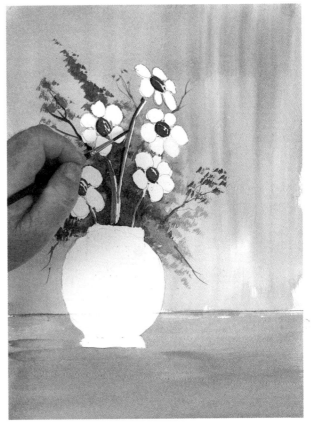

Now we come to the stems which are painted dark green on the left hand side only. So paint the stems dark green on the left using equal amounts of Raw Sienna and Burnt Umber.

To paint the vase we use the small brush and a mixture of Burnt Umber and Light Red.

You will notice that the vase is much darker on the left than it is on the right.

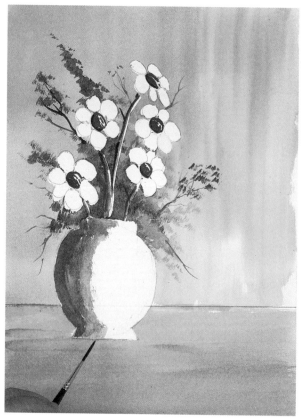

This is achieved by starting with a darker mixture on the left, in other words more Burnt Umber in the mixture and as you move over towards the right use less Burnt Umber and more water until eventually almost clear water.

This gives the impression that it's a nice bright day outside and the sun is shining on the bowl.

So starting on the left hand side, paint the vase. As you go across the vase lighten the colour by adding more water. Paint the vase in the direction of its shape. In this case the vase is rounded, so paint rounded strokes.

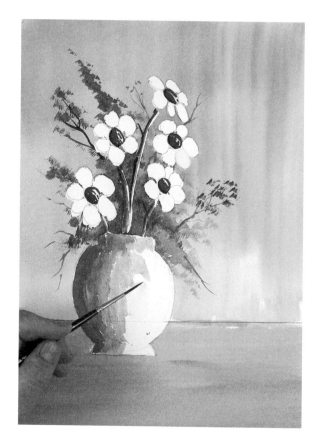

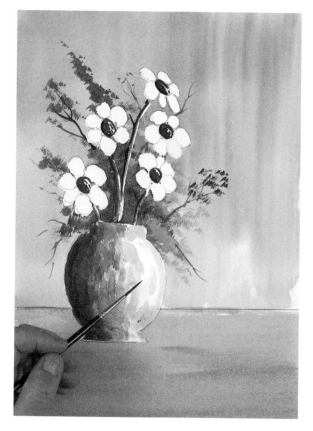

The neck of the vase looks a little naked so let's put some finishing touches around the vase. Once more take the large brush out of the water and dry it on the cloth. Then make a green colour for more foliage using Lemon Yellow Hue and Cobalt Blue Hue. Add a little green around the top of the vase with the corner of the large brush.

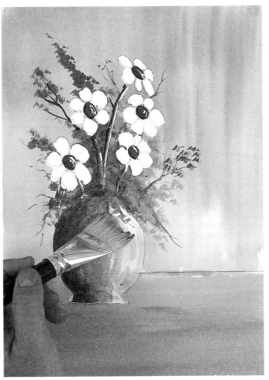

Step 4: Fun - Foreground

On the left there is a shadow behind the vase. So with the small brush, mix some Alizarin Crimson and Cobalt Blue Hue together to get a nice purple colour.

Use this mixture to paint the shadow of the vase.

Tip: Be careful, don't overdo the shadow by making it too big

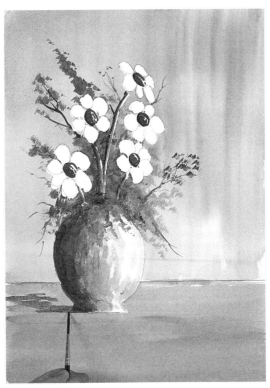

125

Some of the leaves have fallen off the flowers and are lying around the bottom of the vase.

Using the small brush with green for the leaves and Burnt Umber for brown twigs, paint a few pieces of debris around the bottom of the vase.

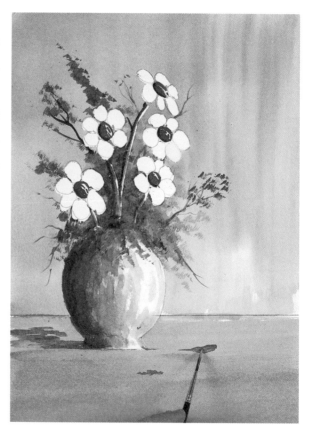

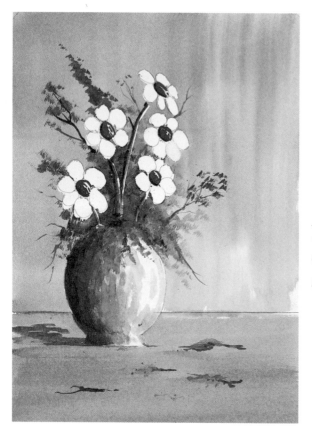

Now I am going to paint my bird, you don't need to, it just happens to be something I do with every picture.

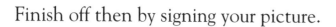

Finish off then by signing your picture.

Tip: When signing a still life it's a good idea to sign it higher in the picture rather than at the bottom.

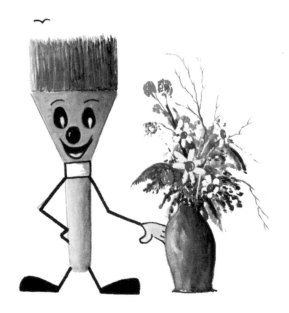

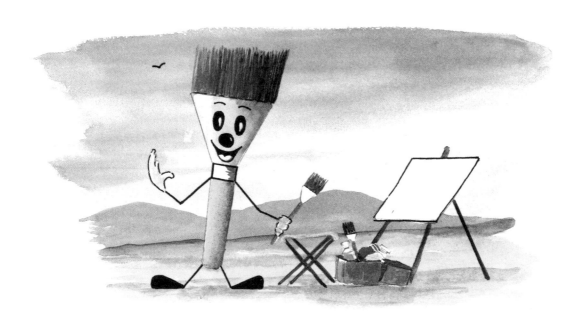

Dear Reader,

Well that completes another watercolour book which I do hope you have used and enjoyed.

You know, if you don't try something you will never realise your potential A wise man once said, 'the best artists never painted a picture because they never tried'. Sad to say many people say to me 'Frank I read your book and I am going to try it out when I get the chance'. There is no time like now and to say 'I haven't got the time' is no excuse. You can make time and when you do I promise you will have a hobby for life.

You must forgive me if I seem to be preaching but the fact is, I so strongly believe in your ability to **Have Some More Fun** painting that I ask you to please, please try it out, you won't be sorry.

I am afraid that art suffers from elitism, this disease causes people who suffer from it to believe that art is only for the chosen few and the rest of us are unable to grasp or understand it. The funny thing is that many of these people don't paint, write or sculpt themselves, so don't be put off.

Remember art is for everyone. This wonderful hobby has changed my life for the better and I promise it can change yours too.

Till we meet again, goodbye from Mr. Brush and myself.

Have Some More Fun

Frank Clarke

Videos

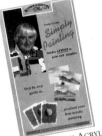

INTRODUCTORY ACRYLIC
VIDEO
SIMPLY PAINTING PRODUCT CODE AHV 001

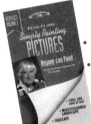

LESSONS
- Still Life
  Bowl of Fruit
- Multicoloured
  Landscape
- Seascape

ACRYLIC VIDEO LESSONS
PICTURES ANYONE CAN PAINT
SIMPLY PAINTING PRODUCT CODE SPAC 123

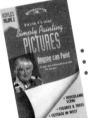

LESSONS
- Woodland Scene
- Figures & Trees
- Cottage in the West

ACRYLIC VIDEO LESSONS
PICTURES ANYONE CAN PAINT
SIMPLY PAINTING PRODUCT CODE SPAC 426

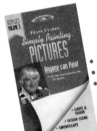

LESSONS
- Light & Shade
- Ocean Scene
- Snowscape

ACRYLIC VIDEO LESSONS
PICTURES ANYONE CAN PAINT
SIMPLY PAINTING PRODUCT CODE SPAC 10212

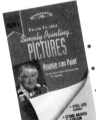

LESSONS
- Still Life
  Flowers
- Stone Bridge &
  Stream
- Historic Landscape

ACRYLIC VIDEO LESSONS
PICTURES ANYONE CAN PAINT
SIMPLY PAINTING PRODUCT CODE SPAC 729

Simply Painting
Acrylic Painting Products

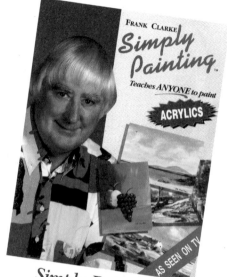

Simply Painting
ACRYLICS BOOK 1
TEACHES ANYONE TO PAINT
ISBN 0951251058
SIMPLY PAINTING PRODUCT CODE ACRBK 01

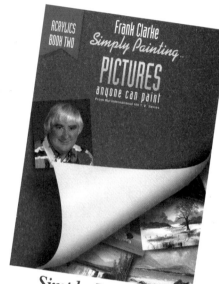

Simply Painting
ACRYLICS BOOK 2
PICTURES ANYONE CAN PAINT
ISBN 0951251074
SIMPLY PAINTING PRODUCT CODE ACRBK 02

Simply Painting **Books and Video**s are available from
P.O. Box 3312 Dublin 6W Ireland
or by telephoning:

Ireland	1850 510 810
UK	0181 938 3545
USA	1800 444 25 24
USA	1800 950 9648

Simply Painting
ACRYLIC PAINTING KIT
SIMPLY PAINTING PRODUCT CODE 219 0719

Frank Clarke *Simply Painting* products are distributed by Winsor & Newton
and available through all Fine Art stores